LIFE enhancement's
5-HTP
archives

by Dr. Gail Valentine
and Will Block

LIVELONG PUBLISHING™
Post Office Box 751390
Petaluma CA 94975-1390

•

FAX (707) 769-8016
www.life-enhancement.com

D1019984

Life Enhancement's
5-HTP Archives
by Dr. Gail Valentine and Will Block

LiveLong Publishing
PO Box 751390
Petaluma Ca 94975-1390
FAX 707 769-8016
www.life-enhancement.com

Library of Congress Card Catalog No.: 98-87054
First printing 1998
Printed in Korea
First edition

Library of Congress Cataloging-in-Publication Data
Valentine, Gail, DO; Block, Will
Life Enhancement's 5-HTP Archives
/ Dr. Gail Valentine and Will Block.
        Includes references and index.
        1. Depression—nutritional aspects
        2. Anxiety—nutritional aspects
        3. Insomnia—nutritional aspects
        4. Weight loss—nutritional aspects
        5. Psychonutrition
        6. Aging—prevention
        7. Health

ISBN: 0-9666430-0-3   9.95

10 9 8 7 6 5 4 3 2 1

ACKNOWLEDGMENTS

We would first like to take this opportunity to acknowledge Durk Pearson and Sandy Shaw as the principal creators and patriarch/matriarch of life extension. Without the actualization of their studies, ideas, and dedication, the whole concept and mission of a new and elevated standard of health, life enhancement, and the global goal of extending lifespan might not exist. We would like to thank Durk and Sandy for their inspiration and influence on the world and all the availability and support that they have given to us personally.

We would like to thank Ward Dean, MD, Jonathan Wright, MD, Don Kleinsek, PhD, and the many others who have contributed to the consciousness of life enhancement and the extension of life as a whole and for all of their contributions to us personally in molding our direction on this life enhancement journey.

We give special acknowledgment to Michael Young and Dale Fowkes whose committed daily efforts make this quest feasible. And we are exceptionally grateful to Paul Dushkind whose dedication made this book possible.

Our gratitude goes out to all the foot soldiers of neuroscience, and especially those researchers who struggle for years to determine what is true about the brain, how it functions, and what we can do to improve it.

If these neuroscientists practically apply the findings of their own research, we suspect they will attain yet higher levels of discovery about life enhancement and life extension — and take us there even faster.

No mention of John Morganthaler.

Disclaimer

Attention readers: The information in this book has been researched, written and presented for educational purposes only. It is not the intention of the authors or editors to provide medical advice. Any application of the information in this book should be under the care of your personal physician. Neither should the information contained in this book be used for self-diagnosis.

"Be careful of reading health books," Mark Twain said. "You might die of a misprint." While we believe that the information contained in this book is accurate, especially compared with other popular health books, we are not infallible. This book could contain errors. Even when working with your personal physician, it is *inadvisable* to rely on this book solely as the source of your information.

It is not our intention to make any recommendations concerning the sources or the amounts or doses of any of the items described in this book. While one of us is a doctor, the information in this book is provided as a starting point. Once again, please consult with your personal physician when attempting to implement any of the ideas contained within.

Table of Contents

Introduction

We have both observed and enthusiastically participated in the **psychonutritional and psychopharmacological revolution (PsyNu Revolution)** which has dramatically changed the psychological health of millions of people in American and progressively around the globe. The **PsyNu Revolution** is unlike anything that has ever taken place. It has radically reduced psychological and physical pain and suffering and helped to cure a wide range of afflictions from mild anxiety on through to suicidal depression. The **PsyNu Revolution** has caused the release of enormous amounts of creative energy directly benefiting those who have gotten relief from nutrients, as well as having given indirect benefits to their loved ones, their coworkers, colleagues, and friends. The tragic veil of a longterm or life sentence of misery has been lifted from many who have suffered the doubts and pains of anxiety, depression, migraine, fibromyalgia, lethargy, and many other ailments. The world is now a better place.

As a medical professional, one of us (physician/editor/author Dr. Gail Valentine) has gained insight from her experience in the clinical arena having studied and prescribed the now dominant selective serotonin reuptake inhibitors (SSRIs) such as Prozac, Paxil, and Zoloft, as well as some of the predecessor tricylcic antidepressants. The use of these drugs comprise a very significant portion of psychopharmacology (**PsyPhar**), the study and administration of drugs that alter psychological behavior. Dr. Valentine has also studied addiction medicine and other psychological pain-avoidance modalities. She is versed in the use of psychonutrients and a strong advocate of psychonutrition (**PsyNu**), the study and use of nutrients and herbs that alter psychological behavior. Dr. Valentine believes that **PsyNu** is a superior and safer alternative to **PsyPhar**. The other editor/author (Will Block) is respectful of **PsyPhar** and has long been a student and researcher of psychonutrition (**PsyNu**).

Typically, **PsyNu** is concerned with nutrient amino acids such as

L-phenylalanine, L-tyrosine, tryptophan and 5-hydroxytryptophan; the former two as precursors to **noradrenaline** and the later two as precursors to **serotonin**. The neuromolecule noradrenaline is the brain's version of adrenaline, the substance that wakes us up and gets us going. Serotonin is the brain's primary inhibitory neuromolecule without which our mind would not be able to take a break.

Together we believe that **PsyNu** is an important alternative or adjunctive therapy as well as a breakthrough, preventive protocol which has been ignored, dismissed, and inadequately "listened to," to paraphrase the popular book on Prozac. It is our aim, with this book, to help rectify this shortfall.

Psychonutritional Self-Help
As members of the boomer generation and thus beneficiaries of the consciousness revolution, we have first hand knowledge about growth strategies which include the use of psychotherapies, the aim of which has been and remains self-improvement and self-enhancement. At the same time, as boomers, we have benefited from and helped foster the exploding interest in alternative health modalities. Individually, it has been a concern of our personal evolutions to research, expound, and to promote the intelligent use of what may be referred to as psychonutritional and psychopharmaceutical self-help. Ensuing this, both of us are proponents of health optimization which we see as an important key to unlocking human potential. However, we are of the opinion that while **PsyPhar** has been of monumental importance in reducing human suffering, the **PsyPhar** approach does not provide a permanent solution and may only be an emergency, temporary remedy. Alternatively, **PsyNu** addresses the root causes of the physiological aspects of optimal nutrition and, ultimately, proper psychological function. **PsyNu** is an active partner, along with volitional choice and self-responsibility, in the achievement of optimal health, both physical and mental.

Our Needs
Fundamentally, we are all very similar in our needs. We all need

water (uncontaminated by toxic substances), oxygen (but not too much), and food (the right kinds, the right components, in the right amounts). We need sleep (to help transfer knowledge into more permanent memory, to quiescence and disarm our emotional buildup, and to rejuvenate our immune systems). We also need shelter, clothing, productive work, recreation, art, leisure, love and self esteem (the feeling that we are worthy of living). When we don't fulfill our basic needs—either not enough or, in some instances, too much! — we tilt the scale against our lives and become unbalanced. This resulting loss of balance hobbles us, limits our achievements and our pleasures, and may even foreshorten our lives. If taken far enough, loss of balance drains that precious essence which constitutes who we are; it pushes us to the edge of the abyss. It is the premise of **PsyNu** that balance is necessary for the proper function of the mind.

Biochemical Factory

Critical to balancing our mind is one of our most important biochemical needs; the synthesis, in adequate amounts, of a natural and necessary regulatory and modulatory brain chemical called **serotonin**. The molecule, serotonin, is also a neurotransmitter, which means it sends messages from brain cell to brain cell. Humans are biochemical factories, and like industrial factories the needs of our bodies are very specific. Scientists have discovered that many of the materials of life are essential or conditionally essential. This means that without adequate amounts of these material foods — as found in the chemicals of plants and animals — we cannot produce the regulating and modulating biochemicals we need to sustain a fulfilling life. We need the right foods — comprised of the right chemicals — to make enough of the neurochemicals, such as serotonin, to achieve fulfillment.

"Natural" Traps

Unfortunately, when searching for the right ingredients in foods for our biochemical factory there are a lot of complexities. First, sufficient amounts are difficult if not impossible to obtain without having to eat too much food and consume too many calories.

Second, *natural* does not necessarily mean that something is good or healthful. In fact, many modern foods have only been domesticated for a few thousand years, and may be quite *unnatural* or foreign to the body (xenobiotic). In their current form, these foods have not been in the human diet until recently.

Grain was first cultivated only about 7,000 to 8,000 years ago in Mesopotamia and much of it was contaminated with fungi even in its natural state. Even today, wheat and other popularly consumed grains are the source of countless allergies. Some popular foods such as tomatoes have been eaten for only several hundred years and many people are allergic to the entire tomato family (nightshades). With regard to meat, poultry and fish, more adoptability has occurred, although the fat content of farm-raised animals and fish is many multiples the level of the wild animals that our ancestors knew. Therefore, it is false to believe that because foods are called natural, they are necessarily good for us and can satisfy our biochemical needs.

Co-Evolution?

Another presumption made about natural food is that it is wholesome. This is far from accurate. As toxicologist Bruce Ames has pointed out, plants naturally make about 10,000 times the amount of pesticides that humans make in factories, and these natural pesticides are equally as harmful as the man-made variety. Worse, they are inescapable because they are naturally present in the plant. Plants make many other compounds that are problematic for humans. These may be substances that are naturally carcinogenic (such as parsley, rhubarb, peppercorns, sprouts, etc), mutagenic, or too highly concentrated in certain minerals or vitamins or toxins (for example; seaweed, animal liver, and comfrey). Organic may not mean that something is necessarily good either. In fact, it could mean that the vegetable or fruit is more likely to contain harmful bacteria or fungi because its defense mechanisms are inadequate, not being bolstered by added antioxidants or other protective substances.

There is still another issue some people raise regarding food. If food co-evolved with other life forms to optimize life, because most of our ancestors lived only a short time—20 to 30 years—how could food have co-evolved to optimize lifespan? The idea that food independently evolves to meet the needs of humans is untrue. To the contrary, evolution is the process of competition between life forms. Plants don't want to be eaten any more than animals do. In fact, recently certain plants have been found to produce indigestible enzymes which migrate to the portion of their leaves that are being eaten by pests, in order to "poison" the buggers.

Science to the Rescue

Fortunately, science has found that optimal health, both mental and physical, requires far higher amounts than can be easily gained from foods without subjecting ourselves to too much of what we don't want: too much fat, too many calories, or higher amount of substances that are deleterious to health. Scientists have studied intensively the likely nutrient-candidates for optimal health among the many thousands of biochemicals (20,000 to 40,000 is typical) found in most foods. Some of these components, such as vitamins, hormones, minerals or herbs have been subjected to hundreds, thousands, or even tens of thousands of experiments and have been found to be positive and beneficial for life.

The Right Biochemistry

Of all the biochemical food ingredient precursors and cofactors that scientists have studied, there are those that affect the body and its systems and those that affect the mind and its systems. This book will focus on one highly specialized aspect of the mind (our brain and the central nervous system) which affects our psychology, our well being, and ultimately what we make of our own life. Indirectly, this book is about your brain and it's ability—with the right biochemistry—to exercise consciousness, to choose, to decide, and to judge. Only by biochemically staffing our brains with an abundance of the right nutrients in the right ratios can we referee what goes on in our internal dialog between reason and feeling on one hand and perception and intuition on the other.

There are countless arguments that we have with ourselves.

Should I do this or that? Should I be more assertive? Should I be more humble? Should I take charge? Should I take orders? When is it better to let reason decide? What are the limitations of operating this way or that way? When do my feelings get heard? What's fair? Who's responsible? How well we do all this is dependant on many things, but at the core of all this is a healthy brain, one which is balanced with all of the excitatory, inhibitory, and motor mechanism neurotransmitters that enable communication throughout the mind and the body at large. A healthy brain also includes many other neurochemicals, including neuromodulators, growth factors, neurohormones, peptides, and on and on.

Take Charge of Your Life
Why is it that some people cannot decide while others have no

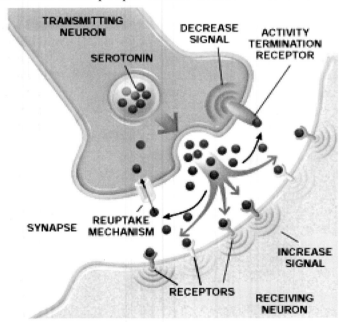

Figure 1. Serotonin release into the synaptic cleft helps to deliver interneuronal messages, but this becomes less emphatic with age as levels of this important neurotransmitter decline. (Meltzer CC et al. Serotonin in aging, late-life depression, and Alzheimer's disease: the emerging role of functional imaging. *Neuropsychopharm.* 1998;18:407-430.) 5-HTP may help restore these levels to those of a youthful adult.

trouble making up their mind? The answer may surprise you. For most of us, most of the time, the answer is that we don't have a good enough internal referee, to arbitrate, to adjudicate, to buffer and to resolve. Our brain is often like a boxing match in which the referee has been knocked out, so there's no one to call the fight, no one to say "fair" or "unfair," no one to negotiate or discern the opposing feelings and thoughts: "yes I must" vs "no I shouldn't."

For many of us life is just that way; there is no qualified or fair moderator and nothing can be done. This sense of unfairness leads directly to defeat. Our response to defeat is the basis of whether we develops the "can do" attitude and the feeling of exhilaration to stand up to the challenges of living our lives. To do otherwise is to court depression, to develop a "give-up" attitude.

Metaphorically, what we will concentrate on in this book will hopefully illuminate and assist in the struggle between the different components of ourselves. These are the components that need to be negotiated, that need to be buffered and resolved. In this book, we will tell you how you can increase the odds, dramatically, of taking center stage, of becoming the ring-master of your mind, of resolving the hopelessness, the fear, the anxiety, the headaches, the aches, the pains along with the resulting depression.

This is not a book for mere contemplation; it is a book for action. Hopefully, when you are finished and have acted on the ideas set forth in this work you will be able to more easily:

- Raise the efficiency of your emotional restoration processes
- Stabilize your emotions
- Alleviate anxiety
- Decrease depression
- Increase your spatial intelligence
- Enhance your ability to lose weight
- Improve the quality of your sleep ... and even
- Become a better decision maker

In a word, you will be better able to determine your emotions.

And you will probably find that you have increased aptitudes in one or more of the following roles:

Arbitrator	Intermediary	Moderator
Official	Judge	Peacemaker
Go-between	Mediator	Liaison
Adjudicator	Negotiator	Communicator
Listener	Umpire	Advisor

Biochemistry Matters

Now wait a minute! If what we're saying is true or even partially true, this is the one-in-one-hundred self-help book to make up for all of the others. All those self-help books promised you the moon and delivered not so much as a morsel of green cheese. The difference between all those others and this one is that the findings of science stands squarely with our premise that biochemistry matters, the idea of this book. Through tens of thousands of articles in the scientific literature, the same theme is apparent. Evolution has created within us the mechanisms to help fulfill our needs as judges, as moderators, and as decision makers. The key to this mastery, is a molecule which we make endogenously, within ourselves. Yet it is a molecule principally used only by higher life forms. It is a molecule that is input dependant on the right raw materials in the form of foods or food supplements. This molecule is serotonin.

Replacing adequate amounts of this molecule as deficiencies arise can tame violent prisoners, soothe neurotics, appease bipolar depressants, and make garden-variety dysfunctionals into producers, achievers and happy campers. Frequently, serotonin deficiency can cause subtler symptoms: there may be days that are just not as alive as they once were; you may have problems with sleep, anxiety, loss of energy, feelings of fatigue, and sometimes even feel hopeless. Taking supplements to restore adequate levels of the neurotransmitter serotonin can make all the difference helping to shift us from dysfunctionality and depression to aliveness and joy.

Dr. Gail Valentine
Will Block
Petaluma, California
Summer, 1998

CHAPTER 1

Depression, Anxiety & Sleep Breakthrough

"With all due deference to scientific scepticism, the reluctance shown by some authors ... to concede 5-HTP its place among acknowledged pharmacotherapeutics routinely applied against depression does not seem warranted, neither on empirical nor on theoretical grounds."
—W. Pöldinger, B. Calanchini, & W. Schwarz
Authors of a 1991 review published in Psychopathology

We are living in the age of Prozac, Zoloft, Paxil, and other similar drugs. Originally developed to treat depression, these drugs are now also widely prescribed for such disorders as anxiety, obsessive-compulsive disorder, migraine headaches, sleep disturbances, weight loss, PMS, obesity, and back pain. Not only do we take these drugs, we also "listen" to them. In his best-selling book, *Listening to Prozac,* psychiatrist Peter D. Kramer, MD, has argued that taking Prozac and similar drugs may actually help some people reconfigure their personality. This has opened a broad new avenue of use by people with no obvious psychiatric illness, who just want to feel more confident, popular, mentally nimble, and emotionally resilient.[1]

However, taking these expensive prescription drugs may not be the only way to obtain their substantial benefits. Prozac, as well as its chemical cousins, work by increasing the availability of the essential neurotransmitter *serotonin,* or *5-hydroxy-tryptamine (5-HT),* in synapses in certain key areas of the brain by blocking their reuptake (See Fig. 1). Because of this action, they are classified as *"selective serotonin reuptake inhibitors,"* or *SSRIs.*

You can also increase the availability of serotonin by taking supplements containing its metabolic precursors, the amino acids *tryptophan* and *5-hydroxytryptophan (5-HTP),* which increase the cell's output of serotonin (5HT). As you can see in Figures 1 and 2, brain cells synthesize 5-HT by a two-step process that begins with tryptophan, which comes from dietary sources. Once taken up into a cell, tryptophan is converted into 5-HTP, which, in turn, is converted to 5-HT.

Tryptophan supplements have a long history of use for treating

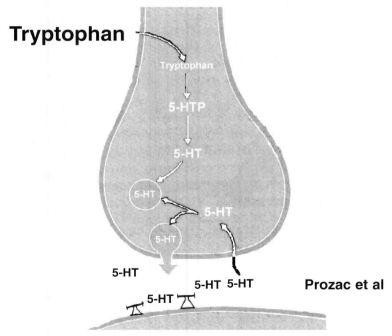

Figure 1: Serotonin Metabolism, Synaptic Release, and Reuptake Inhibition

depression and anxiety disorders, and for enhancing sleep. Unfortunately, since 1988, the FDA has enforced a dubious state of near-total tryptophan prohibition based on the occurrence of serious side effects traced to a single contaminated batch of the amino acid produced by a Japanese company during the late 1980s. This company had altered the time-honored manufacturing procedure for tryptophan, introducing a new and untested procedure while abbreviating an important filtering step.

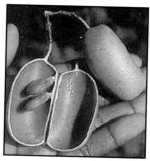

Seed pods from the Griffonia simplicifolia, a West African medicinal plant from which 5-HTP is naturally derived. The bark is antiseptic, the leaf juice is used to treat kidney disease, and other components help inhibit vomiting, diarrhea, and constipation. Griffonia is even regarded as an aphrodisiac.

Such adverse effects have never been linked to any other batches of tryptophan. Nevertheless, the FDA, has maintained its prohibition in the face of overwhelming evidence that it is not only unnecessary, but may be forcing people to take dangerous and expensive drugs to achieve the benefits they could achieve safely and inexpensively with tryptophan.

Fortunately, the FDA's prohibition does not apply to the next step in serotonin metabolism, 5-HTP, though. And while tryptophan prohibition may be needless and deplorable, it has had one unforeseen benefit. It has allowed us to focus on 5-HTP, which, it turns out, may be even better than tryptophan ever was for treating disorders that appear to be related to a deficiency of serotonin in the brain.

The 5-HTP-Depression Connection

Various behavioral and biochemical studies have shown that 5-HTP is closely involved in depressive disorders. In a study employing *positron-emission tomography* (PET) scanning, eight healthy volunteers and six people diagnosed with major depression received infusions of radiolabelled 5-HTP. The researchers found that significantly less 5-HTP crossed the blood-brain barrier into the brains of the depressed subjects than into the brains of

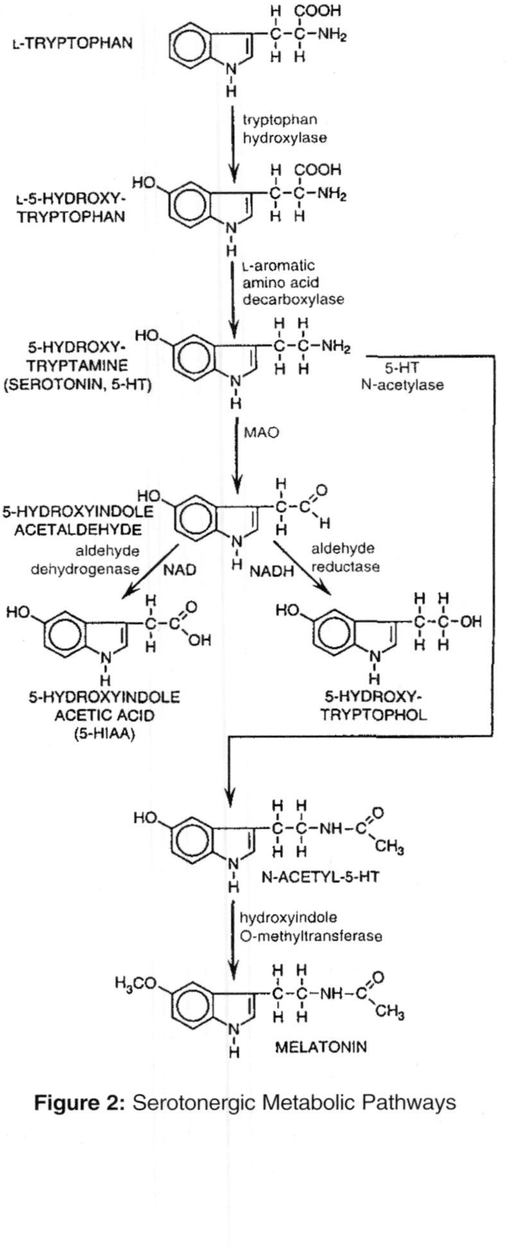

Figure 2: Serotonergic Metabolic Pathways

the normal controls. The authors suggested that the transport of 5-HTP across the blood-brain barrier may be compromised in major depression.[2]

In a French trial of 36 patients with severe depression who were treated with 5-HTP, the authors reported 28 positive results, four cases of intolerance to the treatment, and four treatment failures.[3] Japanese researchers gave 5-HTP to 24 patients hospitalized for depression. After 2 weeks of treatment, they observed a "marked amelioration of depressive symptoms" in seven patients with unipolar depression. The administration of 5-HTP was also found to be associated with a 30% increase in the levels of 5-HIAA, the primary metabolite of serotonin, in the patients' cerebrospinal fluid. This suggested that the exogenous 5-HTP was being converted to serotonin.[4]

Double-blind clinical trials that compared the efficacy of tryptophan and 5-HTP in people with depression found 5-HTP to be clearly superior.[5] A few studies have also compared 5-HTP with standard tricyclic antidepressants (eg, Elavil)—the most effective drugs for treating depression until the development of the SSRIs—and found 5-HTP to be at least as effective as these drugs in treating very severe depression, with fewer side effects.[6-8]

5-HTP vs SSRIs

How does 5-HTP stand up against the current standard of treatment, the SSRIs? That's the question that was asked in a double-blind, multicenter study by a team of Swiss and German based psychiatric researchers headed by Dr. W. Pöldinger of the Psychiat-rische Universitätsklinik in Basel, Switzerland.[9] The subjects, all of whom were diagnosed with depression, received either 100 mg of 5-HTP three times a day, or 150 mg of fluvoxamine (an SSRI) three times a day. The subjects were evaluated at 0, 2, 4, and 6 weeks, using standard depression rating scales. They also evaluated how they felt.

The results were startling. Both treatment groups showed a significant and nearly equal reduction in depression beginning at week 2 and continuing through week 6. After 4 weeks, 15 of the 36 patients treated with 5-HTP, and 18 of the 33 patients treated

Reduced Depression Scores Following Treatment with 5-HTP or an SSRI

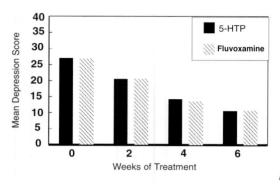

Pöldinger et al, 1991

Figure 3: Mean depression scores (Hamilton Rating Scale for Depression) in patients treated with either 5-HTP or the SSRI fluvoxamine. Differences from baseline (Week 0) are significantly different (*P<0.001*) for both treatments at weeks 2, 4, and 6.

with fluvoxamine had improved by at least 50%, according to scores on the depression rating scales. By week 6, the two groups had about equal numbers showing 50% improvement (see Fig. 3). When the numbers were totaled up at the end of the study, the researchers found that the mean percentage improvement from baseline to the final assessment was actually greater for the patients treated with 5-HTP. The number of treatment failures was also higher in the fluvoxamine group (17%) than in the 5-HTP group (6%), although this difference was not statistically significant. The patients' self-assessments of how they were feeling closely paralleled the scores on the depression rating scales.

Adverse side effects from both treatments were rare and generally mild, usually occurring during the first few days of treatment and then disappearing. Overall, 5-HTP appeared to be better tolerated than the SSRI. Curiously, the *Physicians' Desk Reference* reports serious adverse effects for fluvoxamine in other studies, although no serious side effects could be found for 5-HTP.

Pöldinger and his colleagues argue that, although 5-HTP appears to be treating depression, it may, in fact, be treating a much broader disease, which they term "serotonin deficiency syndrome." This syndrome may manifest in any of a variety of forms, including depression, anxiety, sleeplessness, aggressiveness, agitation, obsessive-compulsive traits, migraines, and other common behavioral disorders; in short, everything that is currently being treated with SSRIs today.

"The behavioral expression [symptoms] of the dimensions related to disturbances of the serotonergic system make up a functional target syndrome, which calls for being corrected through making up for the serotonin deficiency and through inducing a down-regulation of serotonergic receptors," they write.[9] If Dr. Pöldinger and his colleagues are correct about their conceptualization of serotonin deficiency disorders, 5-HTP should also be effective in treating many of the same syndromes that SSRIs are currently used for. While no one has looked at this question systematically, let's see what a brief perusal of the literature reveals:

Relieving Anxiety

Ten patients diagnosed with anxiety syndromes were treated with 5-HTP. A significant reduction in anxiety was observed on three different scales designed to measure anxiety.[10] In a study of 20 people with panic disorders, several experienced a feeling of "relief" after receiving 5-HTP.[11]

Enhancing Sleep

One of the main reasons people used to take tryptophan during the pre-prohibition days was to enhance their sleep. If you look closely at Figure 2, you may see the reason why. One of serotonin's metabolic pathways leads directly to **melatonin,** widely acknowledged today as the hormone that helps determine our sleep-wake cycle. (See article on melatonin, *Life Enhancement News,* Issue 25, p. 7). By increasing your production of serotonin by taking 5-HTP, you're also increasing your production of melatonin. While the role of serotonin and melatonin in sleep has been well-documented, only a few studies have looked at the connection between 5-HTP and sleep. French researchers found that 100 mg of 5-HTP resulted in significant improvement in people described as "mildly insomniac."[12] Looking at sleep patterns in cats, a Norwegian scientist found that 5-HTP had effects on sleep that were similar to those produced by tryptophan.[13]

Suppressing Appetite

SSRIs are commonly prescribed to suppress appetite in people who want to lose weight. It appears that 5-HTP may have a similar effect. A group of Italian researchers reported that 20 obese patients taking 5-HTP (900 mg/day) lost a significant amount of weight, had less carbohydrate intake, and consistently became sated earlier than a similar group taking a placebo. They concluded that since 5-HTP was well-tolerated, it could be safely used to treat obesity.[14] According to British researcher, J. Blundell, of the University of Leeds, of the many appetite suppressants found to be "active" in laboratory animals, very few have clinical potential. Among the most promising candidates, he argues, are those that increase central levels of serotonin.[15]

Preventing Migraine Headaches

Migraine headaches are closely associated with serotonergic activity. The most effective drugs for halting migraine attacks (eg, sumatriptan and dihydroergotamine) block specific serotonin receptors in the brain. SSRIs have also been effective in some people in preventing migraines. A few studies have found that 5-HTP may also be able to prevent migraines. Spanish researchers gave 5-HTP or methysergide, a long-time migraine treatment, to 124 migraineurs. They noted significant improvement in 71% of the 5-HTP-treated people and 75% of the methysergide-treated people. Among those treated with 5-HTP, improvement took the form of reduced headache intensity and duration, while frequency remained unchanged, and 5-HTP caused far fewer side effects than methysergide. The authors suggested that 5-HTP could be a treatment of choice in migraine prophylaxis.[16]

A group of Italian researchers confirmed the prophylactic effect of 5-HTP in 40 patients with migraine in a double-blind study. The patients were randomized to receive either 5-HTP (400 mg/day) or placebo for 2 months. By the end of 2 months, more than 90% of the 5-HTP-treated patients responded with a reduction in headache severity, frequency and duration, compared with only

16% of the placebo-treated patients.[17] In another Italian study, researchers found that administering 5-HTP (5 mg/kg/day) for 3 months to children with either migraine or tension-type headaches resulted in an increase in ß-endorphin and a significant reduction in the frequency and intensity of their headaches.[18]

Listening to 5-HTP

"In functional dimensional parlance, treating a serotonin deficiency is tantamount to treating all symptoms figuring as behavioral expressions of the serotonin-dependent psychological dysfunctions," write Pöldinger, Calanchini, and Schwarz.[9] They point out that these symptoms of serotonin deficiency may include depression, anxiety, sleep disorders, obsessive-compulsive traits, and other psychological disorders. They also argue that the best way to address this deficiency may not be through SSRIs and other powerful, expensive, and in some cases, dangerous drugs. Rather, the answer may lie in a precursor to serotonin, 5-HTP, which has been neglected by many scientists despite tantalizing hints in the scientific literature that it may have profound effects on a variety of extremely common and often debilitating ailments. Perhaps we should be listening.

Depression & Heart Disease: The Serotonin Connection

It is becoming increasingly apparent that psychological depression is a major contributor to heart disease morbidity and mortality, on a par with more familiar risk factors, such as poor diet, lack of exercise, high blood pressure, high stress, and cigarette smoking. This finding suggests the possibility that anything you can do to minimize or eliminate serious depressive episodes, whether using antidepressants or 5-HTP, may also help reduce your risk of suffering a heart attack.

The most recent piece of evidence for this correlation was a study from the Johns Hopkins University School of Hygiene and Public Health. The findings showed that those who experienced even a single major depressive episode (e.g., at least 2 weeks of profound sadness), had a risk factor for heart attack that was more than four times higher than in those with no history of serious depression. This risk was independent of other typical risk factors for heart disease.[19]

Although terms like "a heavy heart," "heartbreak," "heartache," and others have long been used to describe the feelings associated with psychological depression, the link between depression and heart disease goes beyond mere metaphor. The Hopkins study was only the latest in a long line of clinical trials dating back to the mid-1970s:

- In one 1976 study of depressed patients undergoing electroconvulsive ("shock") therapy, both suicide and MI rates were significantly higher in those who were deemed to have been inadequately treated (ie, more depressed).[20]

- In a 1987 study of 50 patients undergoing coronary angiography at the Washington University School of Medicine, 18% were diagnosed with major depression.[21]

- People with heart disease and depression tend to stay depressed longer, which may just worsen their cardiac condition. This connection was revealed by another Washington University study in which 200 patients undergoing diagnostic cardiac catheterization and coronary angiography also underwent a psychiatric diagnostic interview. The researchers found that 17% of the patients were in the midst of a major depressive episode, and another 17% were having a minor depressive episode. In the following 12 months, half the patients with a major depression either remained depressed or relapsed. Nearly half those with minor depression got better, but 42% subsequently became even more depressed. It was concluded that if major depression is left untreated in people with coronary heart disease, it tends to persist. Moreover, people with minor depression are nearly as likely to become seriously depressed as to get better.[22]

- The same Washington University researchers reported that major depression was the best predictor of "major cardiac events" (myocardial infarction, coronary artery bypass surgery, angioplasty, and death) among 52 patients followed for 12 months after cardiac catheterization.[23]

- People with established coronary artery disease have a significantly poorer prognosis if they are also depressed, compared with those who are not depressed, according to a study from Duke University. The researchers studied more than 700 men and women in Denmark, all of whom were born in 1914. They received physical and psychological examinations at age 50 and again at age 60 to establish a baseline. In the ensuing years (up to 1991), 122 (17%) of the participants suffered a heart attack and a total of 290 (40%) died. Those who were seriously depressed at baseline were three times more likely to have a heart attack and to die. The researchers concluded that it was chronic depression, rather than one or more discrete depressive episodes, that was responsible for the increased incidence of heart attacks and death.[24]

- People with clinical depression have a decreased ability to vary their heart rate in response to external and internal stimuli. This relative inflexibility of cardiac function may reduce their chances of surviving coronary artery disease.[25]

- Anxiety and depression may increase the chances of developing high blood pressure (hypertension), according to the results of a large longitudinal study based on data from the National Health and Nutrition Examination I (NHANES-I) Epidemiologic Follow-up Study. The researchers followed 2992 people, who initially had no signs of hypertension, for 7 to 16 years. Baseline levels of anxiety and depression were assessed using standard psychological tests. At the conclusion of the study, it was clear that people who were anxious or depressed stood a greater chance of developing high blood pressure, and that this was even more of a risk for blacks than for whites.[26]

- High job stress may increase your risk of an MI or stroke by making it easier for your blood to clot. Using a group of 22 Israeli accountants as subjects, researchers tested the ability of the men's blood to coagulate on numerous occasions, both during a high-stress tax season and during a more relaxing, low-stress period. Several coagulation factors were found to be significantly elevated during the high-stress season but not during the low-stress season.[27]

Raising Serotonin Levels

If depression is a disease of the psychological "heart," given the link between depression and cardiovascular disease, one can't help wondering whether antidepressant therapy, ranging from SSRIs to 5-HTP, might be capable of alleviating the morbidity and mortality associated with the diseases of the physical heart as well. Such a conclusion would not be surprising, given the proposal that all the disorders that are treatable by enhancing serotonin function, ranging from depression and anxiety to migraine, obesity, insomnia, and heart disease, may all be different aspects of a broad-based *serotonin deficiency syndrome* (SDS).[9] It is very common for some or all of the symptoms of the above disorders to cluster in a single person. How SDS manifests in a given individual may depend on other neurochemical conditions, or it may depend on their personality or other environmental factors. The most likely scenario is that some or all of these conditions and factors contribute.

References
1. Kramer PD. *Listening to Prozac*. New York: Viking; 1993.
2. Agren H, Reibring L, Hartvig P, et al. Low brain uptake of L-(11C)5-hydroxytryptophan in major depression: A positron emission tomography study on patients and healthy volunteers. *Acta Psychiatr Scand*. 1991;83:449-455.
3. Laboucarie J, Rascol A, Guiraud-Chaumeil B, El-Hage W. La place du 5 hydroxytryptophane levogyre dans les etats depressifs. *Rev Med*. 1977;13:519-524.
4. Takahashi S, Kondo H, Kato N. Effect of L-5-hydroxytryptophan on brain monoamine metabolism and evaluation of its clinical effect in depressed patients. *J Psychiat Res*. 1975;12:177-187.
5. van Praag HM, Lemus C. Monamine precursors in the treatment of psychiatric disorders. In: Wurtman R, Wurtman J, eds. *Food Constituents Affecting Normal and Abnormal Behavior: Nutrition and the Brain*. New York: Raven Press; 1986:80-138.
6. van Praag HM, Van Den Burg W, Bos ERH, Dols LCA. 5-hydroxytryptophan in combination with clomipramine in "therapy-resistant" depression. *Psychopharmacology*. 1974;38:267-269.
7. Nardini M, DeStefano R, Ianuccelli M, Borghesi R, Battistini N. Treatment of depression with l-5-hydroxytryptophan combined with chlorimipramine: A double-blind study. *J Clin Pharmacol Res*. 1983;3:239-250.
8. Angst J, Woggon B, Schoopf J. The treatment of depression with l-5-hydroxytryptophan versus imipramine: Results of two open and one double-blind study. *Arch Psychiatr Nervenkr*. 1977;224:175-186.
9. Pöldinger W, Calanchini B, Schwarz W. A functional-dimensional approach to depression: serotonin deficiency as a target syndrome in a comparison

of 5-hydroxytryptophan and fluvoxamine. *Psychopathology.* 1991;24:53-81.

10. Kahn RS, Westenberg HGM. L-5-Hydroxytryptophan in the treatment of anxiety disorders. *J Affect Disord.* 1985;8:197-200.

11. Den Boer JA, Westenberg HGM. Behavioral, neuroendocrine, and biochemical effects of 5- hydroxytryptophan administration in panic disorder. *Psychiatry Res.* 1990;31:267-278.

12. Soulairac A, Lambinet H. Action du 5-hydroxytryptophane, precurseur de la serotonine, sur les troubles du sommeil. *Ann Med-Psychol.* 1977;135:792-798.

13. Ursin R. The effect of 5-hydroxytryptophan and l-tryptophan on wakefulness and sleep patterns in the cat. *Brain Res.* 1976;106:106-115.

14. Cangiano C, Ceci F, Cascino A, et al. Eating behavior and adherence to dietary prescriptions in obese subjects treated with 5-hydroxytryptophan. *Am J Clin Nutr.* 1992;56:863- 868.

15. Blundell J. Pharmacological approaches to appetite suppression. *Trends Pharmacol.* 1991;12:147-157.

16. Titus F, Davalos A, Alom J, Codina A. 5-Hydroxytryptophan versus methysergide in the prophylaxis of migraine. Randomized clinical trial. *Eur Neurol.* 1986;25:327-329.

17. De Benedittis G, Massei R. 5-HT precursors in migraine prophylaxis: A double-blind crossover study with L-5-hydroxy-tryptophan versus placebo. *Clin J Pain.* 1986;3:123-129.

18. Battistella P, Bordin A, Cernetti R, et al. Beta-endorphin in plasma and monocytes in juvenile headache. *Headache.* 1996;36:91-94.

19. Pratt L, Ford D, Crum R, Armenian H, Gallo J, Eaton W. Depression, psychotropic medication, and risk of myocardial infarction: Prospective data from the Baltimore ECA follow-up. *Circulation.* 1996;94:3123-3129.

20. Avery D, Winokur G. Mortality in depressed patients treated with electroconvulsive therapy and antidepressants. *Arch Gen Psychiatry.* 1976;33:1029-1037.

21. Carney R, Rich M, Tevelde A, Saini J, Clark K, Jaffe A. Major depressive disorder in coronary artery disease. *Am J Cardiol.* 1987;60:1273-1275.

22. Hance C, Carney R, Freedland K, Skala J. Depression in patients with coronary heart disease: A 12-month follow-up. *Gen Hosp Psychiatry.* 1996;18:61-65.

23. Carney R, Rich M, Freedland K, et al. Major depressive disorder predicts cardiac events in patients with coronary artery disease. *Psychosom Med.* 1988;50:723-627.

24. Barefoot J, Schroll M. Symptoms of depression, acute myocardial infarction, and total mortality in a community sample. *Circulation.* 1996;93:1976-1980.

25. Carney R, Saunders R, Freedland K, Stein P, Rich M, Jaffe A. Association of depression with reduced heart rate variability in coronary artery disease. *Am J Cardiol.* 1995;76:562-564.

26. Jonas S, Franks P, Ingram D. Are symptoms of anxiety and depression risk factors for hypertension? *Arch Fam Med.* 1997;6:43-49.

27. Frimerman A, Miller H, Lanaido S, Keren G. Changes in hemostatic function at times of cyclic variation in occupational stress. *Am J Cardiol.* 1997;79:72-75.

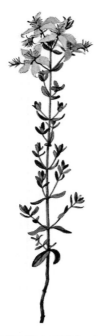

*St. John's Wort is synergistic with 5-HTP
and acts to increase the serotonin-enhancing
effect of 5-HTP.*

CHAPTER 2

5-HTP Synergists and Cofactors:

St. John's Wort and 5-Pyridoxal Phosphate

St. John's wort is an herb that has long been recognized for its safe antidepressive activity, due in part to its weak inhibition of the enzyme monoamine oxidase (MAO),[1] as well as a complex interplay of many constituents.[2]

The scientific literature contains 14 placebo-controlled studies in which St. John's wort was tested in the treatment of depression. One study compared an extract of St. John's wort (supplying approximately 2.0 mg daily of the active ingredient hypericin) with placebo. At the end of the 8-week treatment period, the group taking St. John's wort extract showed a 70% improvement using a standard scale of measurement (Hamilton Depression scale), while the placebo group showed a 45% increase in depression. No adverse reactions were noted in the treatment group.[3]

In another study, 65 patients suffering from mild to moderate depression took 900 mg/day of St. John's wort extract (supplying 2.7 mg of hypericin daily). Another group received placebo. After 6 weeks, the response rate in the St. John's wort group was 67% higher than baseline, compared with a 27% reduction in the placebo group. Two mild adverse reactions were reported in the active medication group — pruritus and fatigue.[4]

St. John's wort outperformed or equaled the antidepressive drugs maprotiline hydrochloride and imipramine in a comparative multicenter study.[5] In this trial, 135 patients with depression were given either St. John's wort (900 mg/day) or imipramine (75 mg/day) for 6 weeks. The St. John's wort-treated group was rated better than imipramine group on the Hamilton scale, and slightly better, although not significantly different, on the two other tests. Adverse reactions were reported in 16% of patients taking imipramine, while only 12% of those taking St. John's wort experienced side effects.[6]

Overall, the incidence of adverse drug reactions related to St. John's wort has varied from 0% to 25% in clinical trials,[7] which is lower than with most prescription antidepressants. Among the most common side effects are emotional vulnerability, fatigue, pruritus, and weight increase. Because St. John's wort may cause photosensitivity, persons with fair skin should avoid exposure to strong sunlight and other sources of ultraviolet light when taking it.[8]

5-Pyridoxal Phosphate

5-Pyridoxal phosphate (a form of vitamin B_6) is a known cofactor in the production of serotonin from 5-HTP. In a study with monkeys, pyridoxine phosphate was found to increase synthesis of serotonin by as much as 60%.[9] Thus it is likely that pyridoxine will help to increase serotonin levels in humans, thereby improving the efficacy of 5-HTP supplementation.

References

1. Reichert RG. St. John's wort for depression. *Quart Rev Nat Med Spring.* 1994:17-18.
2. Holzl J, Demisch L, Gollnik B. Investigations about antidepressive and mood changing effects of Hypericum perforatum. *Planta Med.* 1989;55:643.
3. Reh C, Laux P. Hypericum p; Extrakt bei depressionen p; eine wirksame. *Therapiewoche.* 1992;42:157-681.
4. Schmidt U, Sommer H. Johanneskraut extrakt zur ambulanten therapie der depression. *Fortschr Med.* 1993;111:339-342.
5. Reichert R. St. John's wort extract as a tricyclic medication substitute for mild to moderate depression. *Quart Rev Nat Med Winter.* 1995:275-278.
6. Vorbach EU, Hubner WD, Arnoldt KH. Effectiveness and tolerance of Hypericum extract LI 160 in comparison with imipramine: Randomized double-blind study with 135 outpatients. *J Geriatr Psychiatry Neurol.* 1994;7 (Suppl 1):S19-S23.
7. Ernst E. St. John's wort, an anti-depressant? A systematic, criteria-based review. *Phytomed.* 1995;2:6771.
8. Monograph, Hyperici herba, *Bundesanzeiger,* December 5, 1984.
9. Hartvig P, Lindner KJ, Bjurling P, Langstrom B, Tedroff J. Pyridoxine effect on synthesis rate of serotonin in the monkey brain measured with positron emission tomography. *Neural Trans.* 1995;102:91-97.

CHAPTER 3

5-HTP helps solve ...

The Serotonin Deficiency Syndrome

Every once in a while, there is a paradigm shift in science that forces researchers to zoom out from their narrow focus and take in the big picture. Such a shift may be underway in the treatment of depression and anxiety disorders.

Long viewed as separate but somehow related disorders, results of new studies using the naturally occurring amino acid **5-hydroxytryptophan (5-HTP),** suggests that depression and anxiety, insomnia, being overweight, and even migraines, are all different symptoms of the same illness — a common deficiency in the neurotransmitter serotonin (5-HT). Let's call it serotonin deficiency disorder, or SDS.

How SDS manifests in a given individual may depend on other neurochemical conditions, or it may depend on their personality or other environmental factors. The most likely scenario is all of the above. It is interesting to note, though, that it is very common for some or all of these symptoms to cluster in a single person. People with depression often also have problems with anxiety, insomnia, weight control, and/or headaches.

The Key Study

The concept of a serotonin deficiency syndrome grew out of the work of a group of Swiss and German psychiatric researchers, headed by Dr. W. Pöldinger of the Psychiatrische Universitäts-klinik in Basel, Switzerland.[1] In a key study that led them to propose their paradigm-smashing concept, Pöldinger and his colleagues showed that capsules containing **5-HTP** were as effective as or better than a state-of-the-art antidepressive drug in treating patients with clinical depression. **5-HTP** also caused fewer and less severe side effects. That drug, fluvoxamine, is a member of a class known as selective serotonin reuptake inhibitors (SSRI).

Although both **5-HTP** and SSRIs work their antidepressive magic in different ways, the end product of both is the same, a rise in the amount of serotonin (5-HT) that is available in the synapse. **5-HTP** is an intermediary step in the conversion of tryptophan to 5-HT. Tryptophan is converted to **5-HTP**, and **5-HTP**, in turn, is converted to 5-HT. Just as increasing tryptophan leads to a rise in 5-HT, so does increasing **5-HTP**, but more directly.

SSRIs, by contrast, increase available 5-HT by preventing nerve endings from soaking up recently released 5-HT molecules that have been floating around in the synapse. This soaking up process is known as re-uptake, which explains why the drugs are called "re-uptake inhibitors."

In addition to depression, Pöldinger noted that **5-HTP**, SSRIs, along with other, older types of antidepressants, have been used with some success to treat all the disorders associated with a serotonin deficiency. However, they note that directly supplying new 5-HT molecules — or substitution therapy — is probably a better solution than trying to enhance the recycling of old 5-HT molecules.

On the other hand, direct substitution of 5-HT is not feasible, because most of the amino acid is destroyed before it ever reaches the synapse. "Why not take the closest precursor crossing the blood-brain barrier and let the brain itself do the finishing step?" they ask.[1] Two precursors of serotonin readily lend themselves to this purpose, tryptophan and **5-HTP**.

5-HTP vs Tryptophan

Tryptophan has been used for years to treat anxiety and depressive disorders, but it has two major problems. First, many of the clinical results from tryptophan are ambiguous, possibly because its metabolism to 5-HT, when taken by mouth, is problematic, especially due to the lack of several cofactors which are not usually present in the diet in adequate amounts.

Second, of course, you can't get tryptophan any more. Thanks to our benevolent protectors in Bethesda, tryptophan sales have been banned in the US for more than 8 years. The FDA questionably based its tryptophan prohibition on a single contaminated batch of tryptophan produced by a Japanese company in the late 1980s, which was linked to serious illness and even deaths in many people who used it. In order to cut corners, this company altered the time-honored manufacturing procedure for tryptophan and introduced a new and untested procedure while abbreviating an important filtering step.

5-HTP, on the other hand, has produced clear and significant improvements in people with depression and other disorders, and it is legally and readily available. **5-HTP** is a natural product that has never been associated with any serious adverse side effects and does not fall under the tryptophan prohibition.

Pöldinger takes the scientific community to task for ignoring the therapeutic benefits of **5-HTP**. "With all due deference to scientific skepticism shown by some authors of recent textbooks on the subject and by others, to concede **5-HTP** its place among acknowledged pharmacotherapeutics routinely applied against depression does not seem warranted, neither on empirical nor theoretical grounds," they write.[1]

In their study comparing **5-HTP** and the SSRI fluvoxamine in depression, the clinical effects of these two treatments, one an inexpensive, naturally occurring amino acid, and the other an expensive, hi-tech prescription drug, were virtually indistinguishable (Fig. 1).

Pöldinger and colleagues also point out that the action of fluvoxamine (like most SSRIs) is highly specific to serotonin re-uptake, with virtually no activity on noradrenergic (NA) and dopaminergic (DA) (ie, catecholaminergic) activity. The actions of **5-HTP**, however, may be less specific, because it is converted to serotonin not only in serotonergic neurons, but also in dopaminergic and noradrenergic neurons. This means that it can act as a "false transmitter" and stimulate both serotonergic and catecholaminergic neurotransmission, which may explain why **5-HTP** has been found to be superior to both tryptophan and SSRIs as an antidepressant.[2]

If you are bothered by depression, anxiety, insomnia, weight control, or migraines, new data suggest that you may have a deficiency in serotonin. Although many expensive (and dangerous) drugs have been developed to treat these conditions, some of which increase the availability of serotonin, it appears that **5-HTP**, a metabolic precursor to serotonin, may be a safe, natural, and inexpensive solution to these problems.

References
1. Pöldinger W, Calanchini B, Schwarz W. A functional-dimensinal approach to depression: serotonin deficiency as a target syndrome in a comparison of 5-hydroxytryptophan and fluvoxamine. *Psychopathology.* 1991;24:53-81.
2. van Praag HM, Lemus C. Monamine precursors in the treatment of psychiatric disorders. In: Wurtman R, Wurtman J, eds. *Food Constituents Affecting Normal and Abnormal Behavior: Nutrition and the Brain.* New York: Raven Press; 1986:80-138.

CHAPTER 4
5-HTP for Better Memory

5-Hydroxytryptophan (5-HTP) has been found to increase spatial memory in rats. When researchers at Haifa University in Israel gave old rats the serotonergic precursor 5-HTP, the learning problems associated with age-dependent spatial learning deficits were decreased.[1]

Cognitive functions, especially short term and spatial memory, are thought to be seated in the hippocampus area of the brain. When the hippocampus is lesioned (ie, damaged) in rats, their ability to perform certain clearly defined tasks is adversely affected. These rats are no longer able to perform a water maze experiment in which they have to locate and escape to an invisible platform located slightly below the surface of the water. However, lesioning does not affect the ability of these same rats to first locate and then escape to a visible platform in the same maze.[2] Thus, lesioning the hippocampus causes a decline in the spatial memory ability of rats, without affecting their visually-cued memory.

Cholinergic Paradox

It is known that cholinergic functions, such as certain aspects of memory are reduced during aging. Yet when cholinergic deficits are induced in young rats, the behavioral equivalent of aged-related cholinergic deficits does not occur. Thus, scientists have long thought that the reduced function of any single neurotransmitter cannot explain the problem of age-related memory deficits in old rats. By implication, scientists similarly reasoned that the supplementation of any single neurotransmitter's precursors could not alleviate age-related memory deficits.

The hypothesis put forward by the Haifa researchers notes that the serotonergic system in aged rats is also altered. They argue that this decline, in conjunction with a deterioration in cholinergic function, concomitantly (and possibly with synergy) adversely affects memory. In other words, the combined serotonergic and cholinergic reductions of aging are together responsible for the observed neurophysiological/behavioral deficits in aged rats.[3]

Moreover, other studies have demonstrated that neither serotonergic nor cholinergic lesions by themselves impair water maze behavior. However, when areas of activity of both serotonin and choline are lesioned in the hippocampus, severe learning spatial deficits result.[4]

Operating under the assumption that the combined dysfunctions among the serotonergic and cholinergic systems underlie behavioral deficits seen in aged rats, it seemed reasonable to believe that restoring one system should be enough to improve the ability of old rats to perform spatial memory tasks. Yet studies have shown that, while enhancing the cholinergic system brings about some improvement, it is not sufficient.[5]

Young Rats, Too

Looking at the other system, the Haifa researchers first found that the serotonin precursor **5-hydroxytryptophan** (**5-HTP**) could increase the synthesis and releasability of serotonin in the brain.[6] When they treated aged rats with a low dose of **5-HTP**, they noted considerable improvement over controls in the water maze. They also noticed a restoration of the feed-forward mechanism in the double-lesioned aged rats. Feed-forward is the counterpart of feed-back, which helps return a system to homeostasis. Surprisingly, young rats also benefited from low-dose **5-HTP**, although their improvement was not as great as that of the old rats.

In summary, when both serotonergic modulation of hippocampal interneuron activity is reduced and cholinergic modulation in the hippocampus is impaired, the result is cognitive deficits that resemble those seen in aged rats. Concomitantly, serotonin (produced and release-enhanced by **5-HTP**) may act in parallel to the cholinergic mechanisms, whereby the hippocampus is innervated by acetylcholine's direct effect on inhibitory interneurons. As part of this interrelation, serotonin may additionally modulate acetylcholine release as the effects of **5-HTP** are mediated by acetylcholine. Finally, serotonergic innervation of the rat hippocampus plays a major role in regulation of the excitability of the hippocampus and in behavioral functions associated with this structure, such as visual memory, and possibly short term memory. **5-HTP** appears to be a principal key in helping to maintain and restore spatial memory function.

5-HTP for Cognitive Enhancement

Scientists at the University of Kansas Medical Center have put the concept of "depressed memory" clearly on the map. While the idea certainly makes a lot of sense, ie, depression depresses aspects of memory as well as spirit, to date there hasn't been a hard look at the differences in cognitive degeneration in people who are seriously depressed.

Reporting on their recent work in *Neurology,* the researchers analyzed the effects of depression on cognition in Parkinson's disease (PD).[7] That they were able to do this is quite an achievement due to the difficulty of interpreting data from small samples and also because there are so many other variables that accompany depression. They found that a sample of 45 PD patients with depression were significantly more cognitively impaired than a sample of 45 PD patients who were not depressed. While there were overlapping areas of cognitive impairment between the two groups, only the depressed PD group had impaired memory relative to the control group.

When they compared 22 depressed PD patients with 22 Alzheimer's disease (AD) patients, the depressed PD group performed significantly worse on visuo-constructive tasks and marginally worse on conceptualization tasks, while the AD group performed significantly worse on memory tasks. The researchers suggest that depression affects cognition and particularly memory in PD and that this impairment is distinguishable from that associated with AD. The serotonergic precursor 5 hydroxytryptophan (5-HTP) has been found to be effective in dealing with a variety of depressions [see following chart] and has also been shown to enhance memory in lab animals. Those of us concerned with age-related cognitive decline should take note.

References:
1. Richter-Levin G, Segal M. Serotonin, aging and cognitive functions of the hippocampus. *Rev Neurosciences* 1996;7:103-113.
2. Morris RGM, Garrud P, Rawlings JNP, O'Keefe J. Place navigation impaired in rats with hippocampal lesions. *Nature* 1982;297:6861-683.
3. Nilsson OG, Stecker RE, Daszuta A, Bjorklund A. Combined cholinergic and serotonergic denervation of the forebrain produces severe deficits in a spacial learning task in the rat. *Brain Res.* 1988;453:235-246.
4. Dickson CT, Vanderwolf CH. Animal models of human anesthesia and dementia: hippocampal and amygdala ablation compared with serotonergic ad cholinergic blockade in the rat. *Behav Brain Res* 1990;41:215-227.
5. Fischer W, Bjorklund A. NGF improves spatial memory in aged rodents as a function of age. *J Neurosci* 1991;11:1889-1906.
6. Wurtman RJ. Effects of their nutrient precursors on the synthesis and release of serotonin, the catecholamines, and acetylcholine: implications for behavioral disorders. *Clin Neuropharmacol* 1988;11(Suppl 1):s187-s193.
7. Troster AI, Paolo AM, Lyons KE, Glatt SL, Hubble JP, Koller WC. The influence of depression on cognition in Parkinson's disease: A pattern of impairment distinguishable from Alzheimer's disease. *Neurology* 1995;45:672-676.

5-HTP STUDY CHART

STUDY	Amount (mg)	No. Subjects	Duration	Finding (number of subjects benefited)
Laboucarie et al, 1977		36		Depression (28+)
Takahashi et al, 1977	60-300/day	20	4 weeks	Depression (15 +)
Nakajima et al, 1978	150-300/day	59	3 weeks	Depression (40+)
van Praag et al, 1972	200 3000/day	5	21 days	Vital depression: (3+)
van Praag et al, 1979	200 mg/day	20	21 days	Vital depression: (peripheral decarboxylase inhibitor used) (superiority to tricyclic with fewer side effects, 11+)
Nardini et al, 1983	300 mg/day	26	28 days	Depression: superiority to tricyclic with fewer side effects
Angst et al, 1977	200 1200/day	36	20 days	Depression: (peripheral decarboxylase inhibitor used) superiority to tricyclic with fewer side effects
Poldinger et al, 1991	300/day	36	6 weeks	Depression: equality with SSRI
Rousseau et al, 1987	100 mg/day	50	60 days	Depression (3 mg dihydroergocristine used also): (significant improvement, well tolerated)
Kahn et al., 1985		10		Anxiety
den Boer, 1990	60 mg	20	1 time	Panic Disorder (20 +, no worsening, relief)
Soulairac et al, 1977	100 mg/day	12	1 time	Mild insomnia (12+)
Autret et al, 1977	600 mg/day	11	4 weeks	Narcolepsy: (trend toward more night, less day sleep)
Cangiano et al, 1992	900 mg/day	20	12 weeks	Obesity: (Significant weight loss, well tolerated)
Bartlet et al, 1973	200-800 mg/day	25	10-240 days	Melancholia (19+)
Lobez et al, 1976	50-300 mg/day	14	15-20 days	Endogenous depression (12+)
Sano et al, 1972	50-300 mg/day	107	7-35 days	Endogenous depression (74+)
Fujiwara et al, 1974	50-200 mg/day	20	7-28 days	Endogenous depression (10+)
Titus et al, 1986		124		Migraine: Possibly superior to other migraine treatments
De Benedittis et al, 1986	400/day	31	2 months	Migraine (16+)
Bouchard et al, 1986	100-600 mg/day	~	1 month	Depression (Vit B$_6$ given also) (Improvement in mood and better Stage IV slow sleep)
Kaneko et al, 1979	150-300 mg/day	18	1 week	Depression (13+)
Puttini et al, 1992	300 mg/day	50	90 days	Fibromyalgia syndrome (50+)

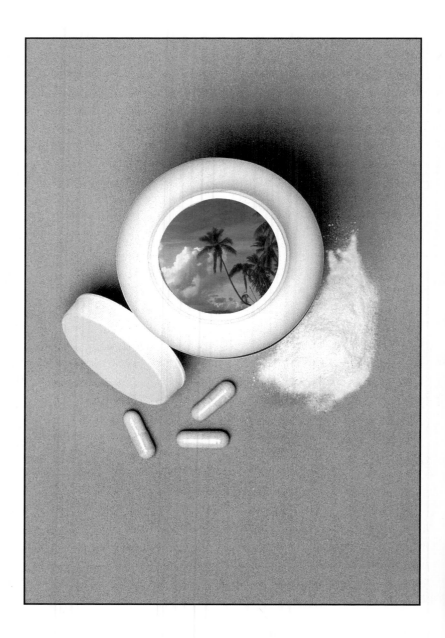

CHAPTER 5

5-HTP and Tryptophan Dependency

SSRI (selective serotonin reuptake inhibitor) users should be reminded that Prozac,® Paxil,® Zoloft® and the rest do not produce any serotonin (5-HT). As a result, tryptophan deficient diets will undoubtedly adversely influence the effect of SSRI drugs. Serotonin is produced from tryptophan in the body. A recent study found that the depletion of tryptophan from the diet has very negative consequences.[1]

When tryptophan-free amino acid mixtures were administered to depressed patients responding to SSRI therapy, their clinical state worsened. This is because insufficient tryptophan availability to the brain results in decreased serotonin synthesis, and thus, less serotonin for SSRIs to act on. **5-hydroxytryptophan (5-HTP)** increases production of serotonin, so this problem, or a variant of it, is far less likely to occur if one is taking **5-HTP**. Moreover, one doesn't have to depend on a tryptophan-rich diet — something not always easy to obtain in these days of fat-phobia and FDA-imposed tryptophan supplement prohibition.

Even if one is not using an SSRI, research has demonstrated that, unless you're getting enough tryptophan in your diet, there is a price to pay. In one study, normal male human subjects ingested amino acid mixtures which were either 1) tryptophan-free, 2) balanced or 3) contained excess tryptophan.[2] The tryptophan-free mixture resulted in rapid (within 5 hours) depletion of plasma tryptophan, and significantly elevated scores on the depression scale of the multiple affect adjective check list.

Tryptophan deprivation also resulted in worse performances than the other two groups in a proofreading task that was carried out while the subjects were listening to a tape with themes of hopelessness and helplessness. (Were they listening to the presidential debates?) Although the mood-lowering effect of tryptophan deprivation was not as great as that seen in depressed patients on tryptophan diets, the researchers suggested that low brain serotonin might be contributing to the precipitation of depression in some patients. Depressed patients might have higher tryptophan requirements which only supplementary tryptophan (or **5-HTP**) can satisfy.

References
1. Bel N, Artigas F. Reduction of serotonergic function in rat brain by tryptophan depletion: Effects in control and fluvoxamine-treated rats. *J Neurochem* 1996;67:669-676.
2. Young SN, Smith SE, Pihl RO, Ervin FR. Tryptophan depletion causes a rapid lowering of mood in normal males. *Psychopharm* 1985;87:173-177.

CHAPTER 6

5-HTP: Misinformation Versus Fact

We've received a few calls lately with questions regarding the safety of L-5 hydroxytryptophan (5-HTP). We decided that the simplest, most complete and most direct way to answer these questions specifically is to do so in a Question and Answer format. What follows is an item by item response to some of the myths floating around:

Q: Does serotonin circulating in the body cross the blood-brain barrier?

A: Not to any significant degree. Because of the size of the serotonin molecule, it cannot readily cross the blood brain barrier. Therefore it is necessary to ensure that adequate levels of serotonin are produced in the brain to prevent serotonin deficiency problems.

Q: Is 5-HTP converted to serotonin (decarboxylated) before it crosses the blood brain barrier? Do we end up with serotonin in the blood and peripheral tissues but not in the brain?

A: Some is, some isn't. Some of the tryptophan in your diet — the "upstream mother precursor" — gets converted to serotonin in the brain, and some becomes serotonin in your blood and peripheral tissues. Studies have shown that 5-HTP taken orally by itself also increases serotonin levels in the brain. And, as is the case with tryptophan, production of serotonin from 5-HTP is divided — some 5-HTP is converted to serotonin in the periphery (before reaching the brain), and some is converted in the brain. Whatever the percentage split, 5-HTP has been shown to compare favorably to Prozac® and other SSRIs for alleviating depression. This is attributed to 5-HTP's ability to increase levels of serotonin in the brain.

. . . .

Q: I understand that when Europeans take 5-HTP, they take it with peripheral decarboxylase inhibitors such as carbidopa or benserazide. Does this mean that carbidopa must be used to get desirable results when taking 5-HTP?

A: No, quite a few studies have been done with 5-HTP in humans in which the 5-HTP was given with nothing else. 5-HTP works as well (if not better) when used without peripheral decarboxylase inhibitors.[1] Moreover, side effects have been found to be greater with peripheral decarboxylase inhibitors than without. A review of the scientific literature found that 5-HTP given alone had better results (249 out of 389 subjects were found improved) than when 5-HTP was used with a peripheral decarboxylase inhibitor (93 out of 176 subjects). This represents a significant superiority of 21% (64% vs 52.9%) for 5-HTP alone over 5-HTP with a peripheral decarboxylase inhibitor.

Q: Does vitamin B_6 cause 5-HTP to rapidly convert into serotonin before it even reaches the brain? Does this mean you don't get an increase of brain serotonin?

A: No, actually quite the opposite. In one notable study on rats, vitamin B_6 deficiency was deliberately induced. It was discovered that very little serotonin was produced in the rat brain when deficient in B_6.[4] In other experiments with monkeys and rats,[5,6] the presence of ample amounts of B_6 — even to the point of "moderate excess" — increased production of serotonin (in the brain) from 5-HTP by amounts up to 60%. Once again, it is clear that 5-HTP raises brain serotonin levels — with or without carbidopa or benserazide, and with or without vitamin B_6. But the evidence indicates that it's better to take 5-HTP without carbidopa or benserazide and with vitamin B_6.

Q: I've heard that the elevation of blood serotonin levels (caused by taking 5-HTP) can cause: coronary artery spasm, abnormal platelet aggregation, and increased risk of death by sudden heart attack.

A: That would certainly be of concern, if it were true. However, we could find nothing in the scientific literature to support these contentions.

Q: I understand people with a particular (and rare) type of serotonin-secreting tumor called hindgut carcinoid, also have various heart problems, such as fibrosis of the endocardium and right heart valves, and heart failure.

A: That's also pretty scary . . . until you consider the fact that these conditions have nothing to do with 5-HTP. This rare disease (carcinoid) is associated with extremely high serotonin levels (much, much higher than are obtainable by taking recommended doses of 5-HTP). It's true that this disease, in a very few instances, is associated with the heart problems mentioned above. However, nobody who has studied carcinoid thoroughly would jump to the conclusion that 5-HTP or another serotonin precursor might cause it! There is no evidence to support an initiatory role for serotonin in hindgut carcinoid or any disease, nor to justify the contention that 5-HTP can cause the kinds of dramatic increases in serum serotonin levels associated with carcinoid tumors. Furthermore, even if 5-HTP caused huge increases in serum serotonin levels — which it has been demonstrated not to do — there is no evidence that this, in itself, would be harmful or that it could increase heart valve problems. In fact, in cats, 5-HTP-induced serotonin production has been found to reduce vulnerability to ventricular fibrillation.[8]

One caution, however, for anyone with this rare type of carcinoid tumor: Since there is a statistical correspondence between serum levels of serotonin and valvular heart disease in some patients with carcinoid tumors (19 out of 604 in the Duke study),[10] it is inadvisable at this time for those with carcinoid cancer to take supplemental 5-HTP.

Q: It has been reported that a tribe of South Sea Islanders gets right heart fibrosis from eating green banana mash because the green bananas poison them with serotonin. Should I be concerned?

A: The story of these South Sea islanders is complex, and nobody is really sure what is going on yet. Yes, it is true that bananas, especially certain types, contain high serotonin levels. But when high serotonin diets have been examined in the literature, elevations of serum serotonin have not been consistent or on the order of that seen in carcinoid patients.[12]

Q: Is 5-HTP safe only if you regularly test your 5-HIAA urine levels and make sure they remain normal?

A: 5-HIAA is a metabolite of serotonin, so this test would tell you if you had high blood levels of serotonin. However, there is no evidence that taking 5-HTP can drive your serotonin levels to the many multiples characteristic of carcinoid patients.

Q: Would aspirin and magnesium reduce the risk of 5-HTP causing a heart attack?

A: Well, aspirin and magnesium will probably reduce your risk of a heart attack in general. But once again, there is no reason to think that 5-HTP might cause a heart attack.

Q: Could some people suffer from a lethal serotonin overload?

A: There is no evidence of this.

Q: What about published studies which indicate that tryptophan does not convert into serotonin in the blood, but 5-HTP does.

A: Most of the tryptophan and only a small part of the 5-HTP in your diet converts to serotonin in your blood. It is estimated that only about 1 to 2% of your total serotonin crosses the blood-brain barrier and enters brain cells.

Q: 5-HTP will not work for most people and could be deadly to others.

A: This is in total contradiction to the vast amount of published data. The studies indicate a very high responsiveness to 5-HTP. And, there is no evidence that 5-HTP has ever been deadly to anyone. Furthermore, there is no theoretical reason for suspecting this. By the way, there are nearly 5,000 papers referencing 5-HTP in the electronically referenced literature.

References

1. Zmilacher K, Battegay R, Gastpar M. L-5-hydroxytryptophan alone and in combination with a peripheral decarboxylase inhibitor in the treatment of depression. *Neuropsychobiology* 1988:20 28-33.

2. Boranic M, Pericic D, Poljak-Blazi M, Sverko V. Suppression of the immune response by drugs interfering with the metabolism of serotonin. *Experientia* 1984;40:1153-1155.

3. Takahashi S. Reduction of blood platelet serotonin levels in manic and depressed patients. *Folia Psychiat Neurol Jap.*1976;30:475-486.

4. Dakshinamurti K, LeBlancq WD, Herchl R, Havlicek V. Nonparallel changes, in brain monoamines of pyridoxine deficient growing rats. *Exp*

Brain Res. 1976;26:355-366.
5. Hartvig P, Lindner KJ, Bjurling P, Langstrom B, Tedroff J. Pyridoxine effect on synthesis rate of serotonin in the monkey brain measured with positron emission tomography. *J Neural Trans* 1995;102:91-97.
6. Dakshinamurti K, Sharma SK, Bonke D. Influence of B vitamins on binding properties of serotonin receptors in the CNS of rats. *Klin Wochenschr* 1990;68:142-145.
7. Siow YL, Dakshinamurti K. Effect of pyridoxine deficiency on aromatic L-amino acid decarboxylase in adult rat brain. *Exp Brain Res* 1985;59:575-581.
8. Lehnert H, Lombardi F, Raeder EA, Lorenzo AV, Verrier RL, Lown B, Wurtman RJ. Increased release of brain serotonin reduces vulnerability to ventricular fibrillation in the cat. *J Cardiovasc Pharmacol* 1987;10:389-397.
9. Robiolio PA, Rigolin VH, Wilson JS, Harrison JK, Sanders LL, Bashore TM, Feldman JM. Carcinoid heart disease: Correlation of high serotonin levels with valvular abnormalities detected by cardiac catheterization and echocardiography. *Circulation* 1995;92:790-795.
10. Jacobsen MB, Nitter-Hauge S, Bryde PE, Hanssen LE. Cardiac manifestations in mid-gut carcinoid disease. *Eur Heart J* 1995;16:263-268.
11. Pierson HF, Meadows GG. Sodium ascorbate enhancement of carbidopa-levodopa methyl ester antitumor activity against pigmented B16 melanoma. *Cancer Res* 1983;43:2047-2051.
12. Hoshino Y, Kaneko M, Takahashi Y et al. Serum serotonin levels of normal subjects in physiological state and stress conditions. From the viewpoint of aging, circadian rhythm, ingestion of diet, physical exercise, sleep deprivation and alcohol ingestion. *Jpn J Psychosom Med* 1979;19:283-293.

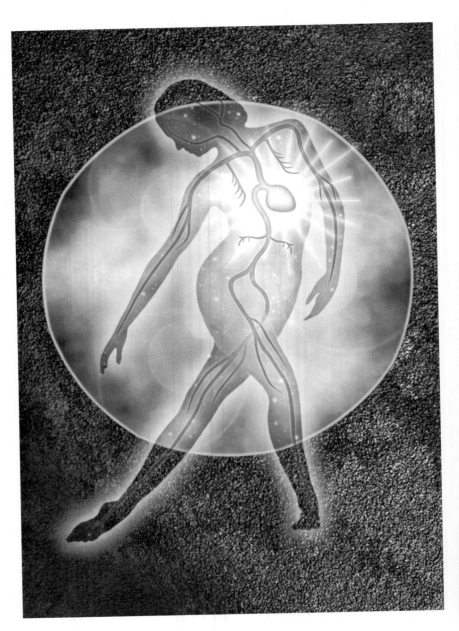

CHAPTER 7

Depression and Heart Disease: The Serotonin Connection

By now we all know the major risk factors that pave the way to a myocardial infarction (MI), better known as a heart attack, include: (1) high blood levels of LDL-cholesterol combined with low levels of HDL-cholesterol; (2) high blood pressure; (3) atherosclerosis; (4) "type A" personality; (5) high-stress lifestyle; and (6) cigarette smoking. And yet there's one risk factor we rarely hear about, even though recent evidence has confirmed that it may increase your chances of suffering an MI some time in your life by more than a factor of four, independent of other risk factors.

That risk factor is depression. According to the results of a new study from researchers at the Johns Hopkins University School of Hygiene and Public Health, if you've ever suffered through a major depressive episode and have a history of dysphoria (two weeks of profound sadness), your odds of having a subsequent heart attack are more than four times higher than if you have no history of serious depression. This risk was independent of other typical risk factors for heart disease.[1]

Although the mechanism by which depression lays the ground-work for a heart attack are unknown, in retrospect, this connection probably comes as no surprise. Expressions like "a heavy heart," "heartbreak," and others have long been used to describe the feelings associated with psychological depression. Nor is the link merely metaphorical. The Hopkins study was the latest in a long line of clinical trials dating back to the mid-1970s that link depression (aka affective disorder) with heart disease. Numerous other studies have also demonstrated a close link between heart disease and depression. Consider these examples:

In one 1976 study of depressed patients undergoing electroconvulsive ("shock") therapy, MI rates were significantly lower compared to depressed patients who were either deemed to have been inadequately treated with antidepressants or who received neither shock therapy nor antidepressants.[2]

If you've ever suffered through a major depressive episode, your odds of having a subsequent heart attack are more than four times higher than if you have no history of serious depression.

In a 1987 study of 50 patients undergoing coronary angiography at the Washington University School of Medicine, 18% were diagnosed with major depression.[3]

People with heart disease and depression tend to stay depressed longer, which may throw them into a downward spiral that just worsens their cardiac condition, concluded another study at the Washington University School of Medicine. Two hundred patients undergoing diagnostic cardiac catheterization and coronary angiography also underwent a psychiatric diagnostic interview. The researchers found that 17% of the patients were diagnosed with a current major depressive episode, and another 17% with a current minor depressive episode. Without treatment for depression, in the following 12 months, half the patients with major depression either remained depressed or — if they improved — relapsed. Nearly half the people with minor depression got better, but 42% subsequently became even more depressed. It was concluded that if major depression is left untreated in people with coronary heart disease, depression tends to persist. Moreover, people with minor untreated depression are nearly as likely to become seriously depressed as to get better.[4]

The same Washington University researchers reported that major depression was the best predictor of "major cardiac events" (MI, coronary artery bypass surgery, angioplasty, and death) among 52 patients followed for 12 months after cardiac catheterization.[5]

People with established coronary artery disease have a significantly poorer prognosis if they are also depressed, compared with those who are not depressed. The researchers from Duke University studied 730 men and women in Denmark who were born in 1914. All received physical and psychological examinations at age 50, and again at age 60, to establish a baseline. In the ensuing years (up to 1991), 17% of the participants suffered a heart attack and a total of 40% died from all causes. Those who were seriously depressed at the initial examination baseline were, significantly, three times more likely to have a heart attack and die. Death due to other causes was also increased by depression but not nearly as much. The researchers concluded that it was chronic persistent depression, rather than occasional depression, that was responsible for the increased risks of heart attack and death.[6]

People with clinical depression have a decreased ability to vary their heart rate in response to internal and external stimuli. Because decreased heart-rate variability is an independent risk factor for mortality in cardiac populations, this relative inflexibility of cardiac function may reduce their chances of surviving coronary artery disease.[7]

Anxiety and depression may increase the chances of developing high blood pressure (hypertension), according to the results of a large longitudinal study based on data from the National Health and Nutrition Examination I (NHANES-I) Epidemiologic Follow-up Study. The researchers followed 2,992 people who initially had no signs of hypertension for 7 to 16 years. Baseline levels of anxiety and depression were assessed using standard psychological tests. At the conclusion of the study, it was clear that people who were anxious or depressed stood a greater chance of developing high blood pressure, and that this was even more of a risk for blacks than for whites (See Figure on page 49).[8]

High job stress may increase your risk of an MI by increasing the tendency of your blood to clot. Using a group of 22 Israeli accountants as subjects, the researchers tested the ability of the men's blood to coagulate on numerous occasions during a high-stress tax season and a more relaxing, low-stress period. Several coagulation factors were found to be significantly elevated during the high-stress season but not during the low-stress season.[9]

Raising Serotonin Levels

These data suggest that depression and anxiety may be as important in the etiology of heart disease as elevated cholesterol — it is oxidized blood lipids and not cholesterol, per se, that causes atherosclerosis — and they raise some interesting speculations about the treatment of heart disease, not to mention the treatment of depression. It seems likely, for example, that people with heart disease may benefit as much from an antidepressant as from anticholesterol or antioxidative agents. Curiously, there is even some evidence that depression can have immunosuppressive effects that reduce killer-cell activity.[10] Perhaps the field of psychoimmunity will find that depression impedes endogenous antioxidant activity.

> **Major depression was found to be the best predictor of "major cardiac events" (MI, coronary artery bypass surgery, angioplasty, and death) among 52 patients followed for 12 months after cardiac catheterization.**

The leading antidepressants available today are the selective serotonin reuptake inhibitors (SSRIs). We've all heard their names: Prozac,® Zoloft,® Paxil,® Effexor,® and several others. They've revolutionized the treatment of depression. Could they be the answer to heart disease too?

While SSRIs are certainly effective for reducing depression, they're far from perfect. First, they are expensive hi-tech prescription drugs, and like most drugs, they have their share of unpleasant side effects. Among these — in as many as 30% of men — is an annoying tendency to depress the sex drive. According to popular medical writer Dr. Andrew Weil, who has a reputation for listening to his patients, "Women are probably equally affected, but there's so much less information available on their experience, possibly because their doctors don't ask questions."[11]

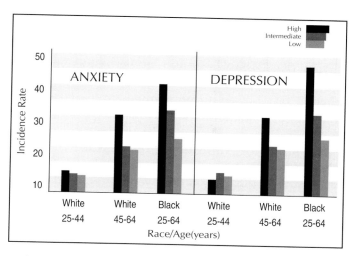

It may be possible to improve sexual desire by lowering the SSRI dose or by taking "drug holidays." These options carry their own dangers, though, including a possible return of depression and withdrawal symptoms.

A better, more natural alternative to SSRIs may be a metabolic precursor to the neurotransmitter serotonin. Here's the rationale: Depression occurs, at least in part, be-

> **It seems likely that people with heart disease may benefit as much from an antidepressant as from an anticholesterol agent.**

cause of a relative lack of serotonin in certain crucial synapses in the brain. SSRIs help by blocking the "reuptake" of serotonin molecules that have been released into the synapse. This effectively increases the amount of serotonin available to stimulate serotonin receptors.

You can also increase the amount of serotonin in a synapse by supplying more of the raw materials for endogenous manufacturing of serotonin. These raw materials include the metabolic precursors L-tryptophan and 5-hydroxytryptophan (5-HTP), which the body uses to make 5-hydroxytryptamine (5-HT), otherwise known as serotonin.

Depleting tryptophan by putting people on an experimental tryptophan-free diet has been shown to induce depression.[12] Both tryptophan and 5-HTP have been shown in numerous clinical trials to be effective for alleviating depression.[13-20] Until it became the subject of a questionable — and unwarranted — government-imposed prohibition in the late 1980s (due to a single batch of contaminated product with one manufacturer), L-tryptophan was the leading natural antidepressant available.

5-HTP: The Superior Natural Antidepressant

Fortunately, 5-HTP, which does not fall under the government's tryptophan prohibition, may be an even better antidepressant than L-tryptophan. In one double-blind clinical trial comparing 5-HTP and L-tryptophan head-to-head in people with depression, 5-HTP was found to be clearly superior.[20]

5-HTP has been found to be more effective as an antidepressant than tricyclic drugs and at least as effective as an SSRI (fluvoxamine).

5-HTP has also been found to be more effective as an antidepressant than tricyclic drugs (e.g., Elavil),® which were considered the standard of care before the SSRIs came along.[14,16,19] And even better, when 5-HTP was compared head-to-head with an SSRI (fluvoxamine), it was found to be at least as effective, and produced fewer side effects.[17]

In addition to relieving depression, 5-HTP also has a number of other advantages for people at risk for heart disease:

5-HTP may help relieve anxiety. As noted above, anxiety is a major factor in the etiology of heart disease, perhaps even promoting the formation of blood clots. Studies in people with anxiety syndromes[19] and panic disorder[22] have demonstrated that 5-HTP can have important benefits.

5-HTP may improve sleep. Anxiety and depression are closely associated (and often magnified) by sleeplessness. To the extent that you can improve your sleep, you can minimize some of the physiological and psychological effects of anxiety and depression. Tryptophan has long been used as a sleep aid, and evidence suggests that 5-HTP may be effective as well.[23,24]

5-HTP may help suppress appetite. Being overweight is a primary risk factor for heart disease. It is also one of the most difficult to control. SSRIs are widely prescribed for appetite control, and now several studies have shown that 5-HTP is also effective.[25,26]

If depression is a disease of the psychological "heart," given the link between depression and cardiovascular disease, one can't help but wonder whether antidepressant therapy, ranging from SSRIs to 5-HTP, may be capable of alleviating the morbidity and mortality associated with diseases of the physical heart as well.

Virtually no research has been published on this important subject, although it is clear people have been thinking along those lines. As already described, as far back as 1976 Avery and Winokur[2] noted fewer heart attacks (and suicides) in severely depressed patients who received adequate electroshock therapy compared to those receiving inadequate antidepressive treatment.

In 1995, a group of German researchers studying lithium treatment in depressed patients also made a connection to heart disease: "Our findings cannot prove definitively that long-term lithium treatment counteracts factors responsible for the excess suicide and cardiovascular mortality of affective disorders. However, our observations are compatible with such a notion."[27]

We will be following the scientific literature closely, because it seems to be only a matter of time before we come across a study with a title like: "Antidepressive Therapy Improves Outcome in Patients with Coronary Heart Disease and Hypertension." In the meantime, supplementing with 5-HTP to avoid serotonin-deficiency syndrome can help dissipate the depressive effect of finding out that you could have done something in advance to improve your outcome for continued health.

References

1. Pratt LA, Ford DE, Crum RM, Armenian HK, Gallo JJ, Eaton WW. Depression, psychotropic medication, and risk of myocardial infarction: Prospective data from the Baltimore ECA follow-up. *Circulation.* 1996;94:3123–3129.
2. Avery D, Winokur G. Mortality in depressed patients treated with electroconvulsive therapy and antidepressants. *Arch Gen Psychiatry.* 1976;33:1029–1037.
3. Carney RM, Rich MW, Tevelde A, Saini J, Clark K, Jaffe AS. Major depres-

sive disorder in coronary artery disease. *Am J Cardiol.* 1987;60:1273–1275.

4. Hance C, Carney RM, Freedland KE, Skala J. Depression in patients with coronary heart disease: A 12-month follow-up. *Gen Hosp Psychiatry.* 1996;18:61–65.
5. Carney RM, Rich MW, Freedland KE, et al. Major depressive disorder predicts cardiac events in patients with coronary artery disease. *Psychosom Med.* 1988;50:723–627.
6. Barefoot JC, Schroll M. Symptoms of depression, acute myocardial infarction, and total mortality in a community sample. *Circulation.* 1996;93:1976–1980.
7. Carney RM, Saunders RD, Freedland KE, Stein P, Rich MW, Jaffe AS. Association of depression with reduced heart rate variability in coronary artery disease. *Am J Cardiol.* 1995;76:562–564.
8. Jonas SJ, Franks P, Ingram DD. Are symptoms of anxiety and depression risk factors for hypertension? *Arch Fam Med.* 1997;6:43–49.
9. Frimerman A, et al. *Am J Cardiol.* 1997;79:72–75.
10. Irwin M, Daniels M, Bloom ET, Weiner H. Life events, depression, and natural killer cell activity. *Psychopharmacol Bull.* 1986;22:1093–1096.
11. Weil A. Are drugs ruining your libido? http://www.hotwired.com/drweil/97/06/ qanda2a.html: *Hot Wired;* 1997.
12. Neumeister A, Praschak-Reider N, Hebelman B, Rao M-L, Glück J, Kasper S. Effects of tryptophan depletion on drug-free patients with seasonal affective disorder during a stable response to bright light therapy. *Arch Gen Psychiatry.* 1997;54:133–138.
13. Agren H, Reibring L, Hartvig P, et al. Low brain uptake of L-(11C)5-hydroxytryptophan in major depression: A positron emission tomography study on patients and healthy volunteers. *Acta Psychiatr Scand.* 1991;83:449–455.
14. Angst J, Woggon B, Schoopf J. The treatment of depression with l-5-hydroxytryptophan versus imipramine: Results of two open and one double-blind study. *Arch Psychiatr Nervenkr.* 1977;224:175–186.
15. Laboucarie J, Rascol A, Guiraud-Chaumeil B, El-Hage W. La place du 5-hydroxytryptophane levogyre dans les etats depressifs. *Rev Med.* 1977;13:519–524.
16. Nardini M, DeStefano R, Ianuccelli M, Borghesi R, Battistini N. Treatment of depression with l-5-hydroxytryptophan combined with chlorimipramine: A double-blind study. *J Clin Pharmacol Res.* 1983;3:239–250.
17. Pöldinger W, Calanchini B, Schwarz W. A functional-dimensional approach to depression: serotonin deficiency as a target syndrome in a comparison of 5-hydroxytryptophan and fluvoxamine. *Psychopathology.* 1991;24:53–81.
18. Takahashi S, Kondo H, Kato N. Effect of L-5-hydroxytryptophan on brain monoamine metabolism and evaluation of its clinical effect in depressed patients. *J Psychiat Res.* 1975;12:177–187.
19. van Praag HM, Van Den Burg W, Bos ERH, Dols LCA. 5-hydroxytryptophan in combination with clomipramine in "therapy-resistant" depression. *Psychopharmacology.* 1974;38:267–269.
20. van Praag HM, Lemus C. Monoamine precursors in the treatment of psychiatric disorders. In: Wurtman R, Wurtman J, eds. *Food Constituents*

Affecting Normal and Abnormal Behavior: Nutrition and the Brain. New York: Raven Press; 1986:80–138.

21. Kahn RS, Westenberg HGM. L-5-Hydroxytryptophan in the treatment of anxiety disorders. *J Affect Disord.* 1985;8:197-200.

22. Den Boer JA, Westenberg HGM. Behavioral, neuroendocrine, and biochemical effects of 5 hydroxytryptophan administration in panic disorder. *Psychiatry Res.* 1990;31:267–278.

23. Soulairac A, Lambinet H. Action du 5-hydroxytryptophane, precurseur de la serotonine, sur les troubles du sommeil. *Ann Med-Psychol.* 1977;135:792–798.

24. Ursin R. The effect of 5-hydroxytryptophan and l-tryptophan on wakefulness and sleep patterns in the cat. *Brain Res.* 1976;106:106–115.

25. Cangiano C, Ceci F, Cascino A, et al. Eating behavior and adherence to dietary prescriptions in obese subjects treated with 5-hydroxytryptophan. *Am J Clin Nutr.* 1992;56:863–868.

26. Blundell J. Pharmacological approaches to appetite suppression. *Trends Pharmacol.* 1991;12:147–157.

27. Ahrens B, Muller-Oerlinghausen B, Schou M, et al. Excess cardiovascular and suicide mortality of affective disorders may be reduced by lithium prophylaxis. *J Affect Disord.* 1995;33:67–75.

CHAPTER 8

More Facts About 5-HTP

5-HTP Suppresses Appetite

5-hydroxytryptophan (5-HTP) behaves as an appetite suppressant even if taken at low doses (50-100 mg).[1] To be most effective, 5-HTP should be taken with a low-glycemic carbohydrate, such as fructose, about 45 minutes before meals. 5-HTP is readily converted into serotonin in the brain, which in turn causes the release of cholecystokinin (CCK), the satiety hormone.[2]

References

1. Ju CY, Tsai CT. Serotonergic mechanisms involved in the suppression of feeding by 5-HTP in rats. *Chin J Physiol*. 1995;38:235-240.
2. Martinelli I, Mainini E, Mazzi C. Effect of 5-hydroxytryptophan on the secretion of PRL, GH, TSH and cortisol in obesity. *Minerva Endocrinol*. 1992;17:121-126.

5-HTP Helps Relieve PMS

When converted into serotonin, 5-HTP helps reduce sensitivity to pain. Because pain sensitivity has been found to be one of the principal contributing factors to PMS, 5-HTP can help alleviate irritability, agitation, and other characteristics of PMS.[1]

Reference

1. Sayegh R, Schiff I, Wurtman J, Spiers P, McDermott J, Wurtman R. The effect of a carbohydrate-rich beverage on mood, appetite, and cognitive function in women with premenstrual syndrome. *Obstet Gynecol*. 1995;86:520-528.

5-HTP Enhances SSRI Effects

Depressed patients taking an SSRI (selective serotonin reuptake inhibitor, e.g., Zoloft, Paxil, or Prozac) who had low levels of tryptophan in their diet were found to quickly lapse back into depression.[1] Supplementation with tryptophan restored the antidepressant effects of the SSRI. 5-HTP can produce serotonin more efficiently than tryptophan.

Reference
1. Delgado PL, Miller HL, Salomon RM, et al. Monoamines and the mechanism of antidepressant action: effects of catecholamine depletion on mood of patients treated with antidepressants. *Psychopharmacol Bull.* 1993;29:389-396.

5-HTP for Scoliosis?

Idiopathic scoliosis, a condition known as curvature of the spine, may result from disruption of postural reflex. The neurotransmitter, serotonin, is thought to play a role in maintaining normal postural equilibrium and muscle tone. A recent study had found that 5-hydroxytryptophan (5-HTP), the precursor to serotonin, can have a positive effect on whether scoliosis develops or progresses, especially if melatonin production and release mechanisms are faulty.

When researchers gave injections of 5-HTP or placebo to chickens that had their pineal gland removed, they found that, while scoliosis developed in 100% of the control chickens, it did not develop in 12/40 (30%) of those treated with 5-HTP. The 12 responders had normal spinal development. Out of the 28 chickens that developed curvature, only six were severe and the rest mild. The mild cases did not have curve progression but maintained their wedged vertebrae. 5-HTP proved to be therapeutic by increasing production of serotonin.[1,2]

References
1. Machida M, Miyashita Y, Murai I, Dubousset J, Yamada T, Kimura J. Role of serotonin for scoliotic deformity in pinealectomized chicken. *Spine* 1997;22:1297-1301
2. Machida M, Dubousset J, Imamura Y, Iwaya T, Yamada T, Kimura J. Role of melatonin deficiency in the development of scoliosis in pinealectomised chickens. *J Bone Joint Surg Br* 1995 Jan;77(1):134-138.

5-HTP, Fibromyalgia, and Migraine

Fibromyalgia sufferers are usually subject to migraine headaches. Is there a common mechanism for both these disorders? That is the reasoning of researchers who administered 5-HTP, either alone or with a monoamine oxidase inhibitor (MAOI), or a tricyclic drug to people with fibromyalgia.[1] Only the combination of an MAOI +

5-HTP significantly improved fibromyalgia syndrome. No subject withdrew from the trial due to adverse effects, although some adverse effects were reported, including sleep disturbances, a mild stomachache, and, in two subjects, transient hypertension, which was interpreted as a possible "cheese effect," which is known to occur when people taking an MAOI eat certain foods containing tyrosine. (This was not confirmed however, as the hypertensive episode was associated with very dramatic emotional events.)

The researchers concluded that the combination of MAOIs with 5-HTP increased serotonergic and adrenergic receptors and, simultaneously, increased serotonin levels in the central nervous system resulting in a reduction of the symptoms of migraine. MAOI drugs should only be used under the supervision of a healthcare professional. Other studies have shown that 5-HTP alone at 300 mg/day can improve fibromyalgia[2] and at 400mg/day can improve migraine.[3]

References

1. Nicolodi M, Sicuteri F. Fibromyalgia and migraine, two faces of the same mechanism. Serotonin as the common clue for pathogenesis and therapy. *Adv Exp Med Biol.* 1996;398:373-379.
2. Puttini PS, Caruso I. Primary fibromyalgia syndrome and 5-hydroxy-L-tryptophan: a 90-day open study. *J Int Med Res.* 1992;20:182-189.
3. DeBenedittis G, Massei R. 5-HT precursors in migraine prophylaxis: a double-blind cross-over study with L-5-hydroxytryptophan versus placebo. *Clin J Pain.* 1986;3:123-129.

5-HTP Reduces Juvenile Headaches

A group of 20 juvenile patients suffering from migraine (13 without aura and 7 from episodic tension-type), were given 5-hydroxytryptophan (5-HTP) for three months.[1] Afterward, they were examined for relative serum levels of serotonin and plasma and mononuclear cell concentrations of beta-endorphins. These levels were then compared with those in a control group of headache-free juveniles.

The researchers found significantly lower plasma and mononuclear cell concentrations of beta-endorphin in all the headache patients, compared with the healthy controls. After 5-HTP treatment, serum serotonin and both plasma and mononuclear cell levels of beta-endorphin tended to be higher. In addition, the frequency and intensity of headache attacks were found to be significantly lower than they were at the baseline.

Reference
1. Battistella PA, Bordin A, Cernetti R, Broetto S, Corra S, Piva E, Plebani M. Beta-endorphin in plasma and monocytes in juvenile headache. *Headache* 1996;36:91-94.

5-HTP and Palsy
Two elderly patients with clinically diagnosed progressive supranuclear palsy were given a variety of compounds including amitriptyline (tricyclic antidepressant) and 5-hydroxytryptophan (5-HTP).[1] Both patients showed postural instability and Parkinson's symptoms. They also had symptoms of supranuclear ophthalmoplegia and pseudobulbar palsy.

The drug amitriptyline at 75 mg/day markedly improved horizontal-gaze palsy, as did 5-HTP at 600 mg/day. The results suggest the involvement of impaired serotonergic system in ophthalmoplegia of progressive supranuclear palsy. This study seems to indicate that 5-HTP can alleviate Parkinsonian-like symptoms, which is especially significant since we all would probably become Parkinsonian if we lived long enough — it's just that those who develop Parkinson's disease do so at a younger age.

Reference
1. Yukitake M, Takashima Y, Kurohara K, Matsui M, Kuroda Y. Improvement of ophthalmoplegia by 5-hydroxytryptophan in two cases of progressive supranuclear palsy. *Clin Neurol.* 1996;36:906-908.

5-HTP and Endorphins
The feel-good hormones — beta endorphins — were significantly increased after consumption of 200 mg of 5-hydroxytryptophan (5-HTP) by patients with major depression who had first received dexamethasone.[1] In normal subjects, dexamethasone suppresses adrenocorticotropic hormone (ACTH) and cortisol levels. In depressed subjects, however, dexamethasone does not suppress these hormones, both of which often remain chronically elevated.

These hormone levels are also associated with beta-endorphin elevation.

However, significant increase in beta endorphins occurred only in major, but not minor, depressed subjects. There was a significant and positive relationship between 5-HTP-induced beta-endorphin values and the Hamilton Depression Rating Scale (HDRS) score that were substantially lower, indicating reduced depression.

Reference

1. Maes M, van Gastel A, Ranjan R, Blockx P, Cosyns P, Meltzer HY, Desnyder R. Stimulatory effects of L-5-hydroxytryptophan on postdexamethasone beta-endorphin levels in major depression. *Neuropsychopharm*. 1996;15:340-348.

5-HTP: Better Than Tryptophan

5-HTP enhances serotonin levels better than tryptophan, because it is one step closer to serotonin in the biochemical pathway.[1] There are benefits attributable to 5-HTP in the literature but not apparent for tryptophan.

Reference

1. Quadbeck H, Lehmann E, Tegeler J. Comparison of the antidepressant action of tryptophan, tryptophan/5-hydroxytryptophan combination and nomifensine. *Neuropsychobiology* 1984;11(2):111-115.

CHAPTER 9

Listening to 5-HTP

5-HTP Users Share Their Practical Wisdom

When 5-HTP first hit the market in 1996, it quickly became a best selling product. This was not a big surprise. Since 1989, when the FDA (for reasons only they really understand) embargoed tryptophan, people who depended on this amino acid for relief from depression, insomnia, and anxiety have had nowhere safe to go. For depression they had to resort to expensive, potent, and sometimes dangerous, high-tech drugs like Prozac,® Zoloft® and other SSRIs (selective serotonin reuptake inhibitors) or tricyclic antidepressants, like Elavil.® For sleep, they had to accept Halcion,® Restoril,® and Ambien;® and for anxiety there was Xanax® and Valium.® For those who preferred a natural solution to these common problems, all anyone could do was offer their sympathies.

Virtually overnight, the introduction of 5-HTP changed all that. 5-HTP or 5-hydroxytryptophan, is the next step, following tryptophan, in the synthesis of the neurotransmitter serotonin (5-hydroxytryptamine, 5-HT).

Pöldinger and his colleagues have theorized that a deficiency in serotonin may be at least partly responsible for a whole constellation of physical/psychological symptoms, including depression, anxiety, insomnia, obesity, and migraine headaches. They have termed this, the "serotonin deficiency syndrome." [1]

While SSRIs and other drugs may be quite effective for treating symptoms of serotonin deficiency syndrome, Pöldinger presented data showing that 5-HTP was just as effective, better tolerated, and probably safer, because, like tryptophan, it actually corrected the deficiency, rather than masking it the way these other drugs do. Better still, 5-HTP seemed to be even more effective than tryptophan for these purposes.

And the best news of all: 5-HTP avoids the FDA's tryptophan prohibition. Thus, for those of you who have suffered through the better part of a decade without tryptophan, the introduction of 5-HTP has meant just one thing. Happy days are here again!

Early marketers quickly knew about and were extremely pleased with their customers' response to 5-HTP. Because 5-HTP is such a new option, and because it has so many possible benefits, there was a lot of curiosity as to just how customers were using it and what their experiences had been with it. A poll was conducted via an informal telephone survey of customers who had purchased 5-HTP to find out why they were using it and what their results had been.

By far, the two primary reasons people said they were attracted to 5-HTP were depression and sleep problems. Not surprisingly, many of the customers were former tryptophan users, and several had been using Prozac or other SSRIs for depression.

One customer from Alaska, for example, reported he was taking 5-HTP for seasonal affective disorder (SAD), the depression that sets in during long winter days as a result of too little sunlight. About 1 tablespoon each evening, he said, alleviated the depression he typically feels each winter.

Another customer, who takes a 5-HTP formulation each morning for depression, told us he now "feels great." That sentiment was echoed by another customer, a medical doctor, who also takes it in the morning. He told us it "works wonderfully." He had previously been taking the SSRI Paxil.

A customer, who takes two servings every night for depression, said she feels "lifted and elevated." She used to take tryptophan until it was embargoed, but now feels that 5-HTP "seems to be working very well," with no bad side effects.

Several responders reported that they are taking 5-HTP to help them sleep better. Many of these are also former tryptophan users who said they have been forced into taking everything from Benadryl® to Halcion to help them sleep. One woman said she finds 5-HTP "every bit as good as tryptophan." A number of these customers took both 5-HTP and melatonin in the evening just before going to bed.

A few customers told us that they were taking 5-HTP for cognitive enhancement. Noted one man in his 70s, "Since I've been taking it, I'm thinking clearer, and my memory seems better."

Most people said that they take their 5-HTP in the evening, especially if they are taking it for depression or to help them sleep. However, there were some who take it during the day, apparently with no ill effects. It appears that as long as it doesn't make you sleepy, there's no reason why you can't take it anytime you like.

How much should you be taking? A lot depends on your individual needs and metabolism. Some customers achieved the desired effect with as little as one serving per day, while others reported that they needed as many as six (eg, two servings, three times per day).

Adverse effects were rare. One customer who was taking four servings per day complained of symptoms suggesting too much serotonin (eg, sinus problems, stomach ache, headache). The most common, although infrequent, complaint was a lack of any effect. In many cases, this could be explained by taking too little or taking it for too brief a period (eg, 1 week).

What has your experience been with 5-HTP? We'd love to hear from you. Give us a call or drop us a line by mail or fax. We too will be "listening to 5-HTP" and reporting on the growing body of scientific information about this valuable nutrient tool.

References

1. Pöldinger W, Calanchini B, Schwarz W. A functional-dimensinal approach to depression: serotonin deficiency as a target syndrome in a comparison of 5-hydroxytryptophan and fluvoxamine. *Psychopathology*. 1991;24:53-81.

CHAPTER 10

Weight Loss: 5-HTP and The Gut-Brain Connection

A class of peptides known as cholecystokinins (CCKs) may help to explain some of the benefits of 5-HTP. Consider the range of 5-HTP's properties.

- It can be an anxiolytic (anti-anxiety agent) or an antidepressive.
- It has been found to enhance spatial memory.
- It can even help reduce appetite.

And that's not all. Is there some other mechanism that can explain how 5-HTP can provide so many seemingly diverse benefits? A growing body of research is finding that the CCK peptides, at home in two seemingly disparate areas of the body — the brain (cerebral cortex) and the GI tract — may help us to understand the known virtues of 5-HTP and possibly other not-yet-realized applications.

It is clear that a strong link between 5-HTP and CCKs exists. When 5-HTP increases serotonin production in the brain, CCKs are released in the duodenum, where they operate as hormones. CCKs are also found in the cerebral cortex in high concentrations where they act as neurotransmitters, modulating the activity of dopamine in the mesolimbic dopaminergic pathway.[1]

5-HTP Activates Your "Calorie Counter"

For years scientists have tried to find the "calorie counter" in the brain, the satiety mechanism that tells you when you've had enough to eat. CCKs may provide the answer to that search.

When CCKs are released in response to certain brain mechanisms — eg, the production and release of serotonin resulting from ingestion of amino acids, carbohydrates, tryptophan or 5-HTP — a variety of effects occur, including intestinal and biliary smooth muscle contraction, pancreatic enzyme secretion, trophic effects on gastric and intestinal mucosa, and appetite satisfaction.

Some brain-CCK-receptor studies have shown that this is due to an unusual bioelectric correspondence that occurs via the vagus nerve and then up the spinal cord. It may be through this nervous system conduit that signals are generated via CCK release and sent to the brain, indicating that the gut is full, thank you. A particularly elegant experiment found that when this message was blocked by the removal of the vagus nerve, satiety was not registered.[1]

When CCKs have been injected directly into the hypothalamus in the brain, they exercise a direct influence over satiety, reducing food consumption.[2] When rats were fed 5-HTP, they produced serotonin which increased the inhibitory effects of CCK-8 on food ingestion.[3] This has been found to be true for healthy non-obese humans as well.[4]

Memory Enhancement
CCKs may play a similar effect in memory. Pregnenolone researchers Flood and Morley have shown that rats fed immediately following a learning experience retain their learning better than without the feeding, and that one of the gastrointestinal hormones released is CCK. When CCK is administered peripherally, the result is the same and the learning is enhanced.[5]

As with satiety, vagotomy inhibits this memory-entrainment effect, strongly suggesting the positive role played by the stimulation of the vagus pathways which ascend to the brain. Other studies also indicate that, when the GI hormonal system is activated by the passage of food through the intestines — and the production of certain neurotransmitters, such as serotonin in the brain — memory retention is enhanced. As MIT researcher Richard Wurtman has pointed out, different foods produce different moods and/or states of awareness.[6] In one of his studies, a specially formulated carbohydrate drink, which increased the ratio of tryptophan to other amino acids, resulted in improved memory word recognition. More serotonin means more CCK activity which means better imprinting of new learning.

The anticholinergic drug, scopolamine, will not produce its usual amnesiac effects when rats are pretreated with the cholecystokinin octapeptide (CCK-8), thus demonstrating the preventive aspects of CCK-8.[7] The actions of CCK have been attributed to its interactions with two types of receptors: CCKA and CCKB. While the "A" receptors are located predominately in the periphery, "B" receptors are located predominantly in the brain and spinal cord. Curiously, research indicates that for optimal memory retention there should be a balance between CCKA-mediated facilitative effects and CCKB-mediated inhibitory effects.[8]

The Notes of Anxiety and Depression

Studies suggest that substances that excite (agonists) CCKB receptors may play a role in generating anxiety and those that inhibit CCKB (antagonists) may produce anxiolytic-like actions in animals. CCKB antagonists are also believed to help predict antipsychotic, analgesic, antidepressant, and memory-enhancing effects in man. In 1995, a researcher from the Lilly corporation called for more research into the relationship between CCKs and depression.[9] Lilly is the manufacturer of the best selling selective serotonin reuptake inhibitor (SSRI) Prozac. Do they know something we don't?

References

1. Flood JF, Merbaum MO, Morley JE. The memory enhancing effects of cholecystokinin octapeptide are dependent on an intact stria terminalis. *Neurobiol Learn Mem.* 1995;64:139-145.
2. Hoebel BG. Brain neurotransmitters in food and drug reward. *Am J Clin Nutr* 1985;42(Suppl):1133-1150.
3. Esfahani N, Bednar I, Qureshi GA, Sodersten P. Inhibition of serotonin synthesis attenuates inhibition of ingestive behavior by CCK-8. *Pharm Biochem Behav.* 1995;51:9-12.
4. Stacher G, Bauer H, Steinringer H. Cholecystokinin decreases appetite and activation evoked by stimuli arising from the preparation of a meal in man.

Physiol Behav. 1979;23:325-331.

5. Flood JF, Morley JE. Effects of bombesin and gastrin-releasing peptide on memory processing. *Brain Res.* 1988;460:314-322.

6. Sayegh R, Schiff I, Wurtman J, Spiers P, McDermott J, Wurtman R. The effect of a carbohydrate-rich beverage on mood, appetite, and cognitive function in women with premenstrual syndrome. *Obstet Gynecol.* 1995;86(4 Pt 1):520-528.

7. Itoh S, Takashima A, Katsuura G. Preventive effect of cholecystokinin octapeptide on scopolamine-induced memory impairment in the rat. *Drug Dev Rev.* 1988;12:63-70.

8. Lemaire M, Bohme GA, Piot O, Roques BP, Blanchard JC. CCK-A and CCK-B selective receptor agonists and antagonists modulate olfactory recognition in male rats. *Psychopharm.* 1994;115:435-440.

9. Rasmussen K. Therapeutic potential of cholecystokinin-B antagonists. *Exp Opin Invest Drugs.* 1995;4:4.

CHAPTER 11

WHAT ABOUT THAT 5-HTP SYNERGIST...?
ST. JOHN'S WORT
(HYPERICIN)
FOR DEPRESSION

Newsweek has felt the pulse of the nation and concluded in a front-cover bannered article (May 5, 1997) that the world needs a natural alternative to Prozac® (and other SSRIs). With just one mention each of pregnenolone and 5-hydroxytryptophan (5-HTP), they take up the case for St. John's wort, also known as hypericin. And the case for using hypericin in the treatment of minor depression is good, although not as well substantiated as that for pregnenolone, or better yet, for 5-HTP.

The antiviral aspects of hypericin were first drawn to our attention several years ago because of its reported use by the AIDS

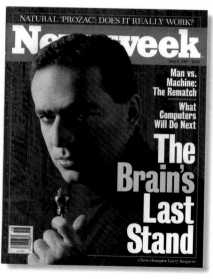

treatment underground.[1] At that time, we saw only the tip of this herbal iceberg. As the most active component in an herb known as St. John's wort, hypericin has been in use for a wide variety of conditions since at least the time of ancient Greece.[2] Among its areas of use are improved wound healing, anti-inflammatory effects,[3] antimicrobial activity,[4] sinusitis relief (perhaps due to its bioflavanoid component, quercetin),[5] seasonal affective disorders, (SAD)[6] and especially depression. Back in the classical Mediterranean world and throughout the folk medicine of the middle ages, St. John's wort's earned its reputation as a powerful mood-altering substance. And now science is confirming this reputation. This property is why some nutrient companies are including a synergistic amount of St. John's wort in their 5-HTP formulations.

Although its antiviral benefits are not in dispute, the very large amounts of hypericin needed to achieve this benefit render the user highly susceptible to ultraviolet excesses.[7] In livestock known to eat large quantities of the St. John's wort plant, there is an increased sensitivity to sunlight, which has resulted in the blistering of skin and even death. This side effect was also observed in a recent clinical trial of hypericin. A few of the subjects had skin rashes and irritation severe enough to prevent them from venturing outdoors. Oddly, light appears necessary for the antiviral benefits.[8]

With smaller amounts, however, hypericin can be quite beneficial and does not require the avoidance of direct sunlight. In Germany, where it is used for depression, it is so popular that over 66 million daily doses were prescribed in 1994.[9] *The British Journal of Medicine* published a review of the treatment literature in 1996.[10] Twenty-three randomized trials of St. John's wort involving a total of 1,757 outpatients with mild to moderately severe depressive disorders were analyzed. The conclusions were quite clear: hypericin was significantly superior to placebo, and seemed to be comparable in effectiveness to standard antidepressants (other than SSRIs) for mild depression. All this occurred with fewer side effects — including impairment of cognitive performance — which has only rarely been observed. Unlike pharmacological antidepressants (5-HTP excluded), hypericin does not lead to any impairment of attention, concentration or reaction.[11]

Many of the controlled studies measuring hypericin's efficacy in depression compared the herb (alone or combined with other plant extracts) with placebo and/or a standard antidepressant.[10] Most trials were double-blinded and lasted from 4 to 8 weeks. The measures used in these studies included improvement in depressive symptoms and evaluation with the commonly used Hamilton

Depression Rating Scale (HAMDS) and the Clinical Global Impressions (CGI) Scale. The daily dose of hypericin varied widely, although the most common amounts were the equivalent of between 100 and 300 mg of 0.3 % extract for a total of 300 to 900 µg per day.

Fifteen of the studies were placebo-controlled (14 testing single preparations and one using a combination with other plant extracts), and 8 compared hypericin with an antidepressive drug (6 testing single preparations and 2 testing combinations).

The most common side effects associated with hypericin were gastrointestinal symptoms, allergy and fatigue. Those taking standard antidepressants were almost twice as likely to encounter severe side effects (35.9% vs. 19.8%). A total of 4% of patients receiving hypericin preparations dropped out of trials because of side effects, as did 7.7% of those receiving standard antidepressants.

In a meta-analysis of the data, the researchers acknowledged the difficulty of drawing conclusions because of the differences in the amounts of the hypericin and other variables. Also complicating matters was the undoubted variation in the contents of the extracts (the same extract was not used in all the studies) and the possibility that other active ingredients were present that fail to show up in a non-standardized extract.

Nevertheless, the meta-analysts found enough evidence to conclude that hypericin is better than placebo in treating some depressive disorders. They could not judge whether hypericin is as good as the standard pharmaceutical antidepressants, although it appears to cause fewer side effects than these drugs. (Hypericin has not been directly compared with 5-HTP.)

In an editorial accompanying the meta-analysis, it was agreed that the data on hypericin are promising but not yet sufficient to accept it as an effective antidepressant preparation.[9] (What else is new?). What is required to understand the efficacy is: 1) dose standardization studies; and 2) longer trials.

How does hypericin work as an antidepressant? Although hypericin is a mild monoamine oxidase (MAO) inhibitor, a recent study found no support for this as an explanation.[12] A more likely, but so far unsubstantiated, hypothesis involves hypericin's relatively strong affinity for gamma-aminobutryic acid receptors ($GABA_a$) an activity attributed to the herb's flavonoid property?[3]

Another explanation posits the vascular relaxation effect of the procanidin fractions of hypericin, which prevents or antagonizes histamine- or prostaglandin-induced arterial contractions.[14]

A final intriguing possibility: In animal studies, hypericin has been shown to enhance the exploratory activity of mice in a novel environment. At the same time, the animals' narcotic-induced sleeping time was significantly prolonged on a dose-dependent basis.[15] As with many — if not most — other antidepressants, hypericin administration decreased aggressiveness in socially isolated male mice.

When researchers and formulators were working on the ingredients of 5-HTP formulation, they were quite aware of the studies on hypericin, which is why they started with the average amount used in the meta-analysis studies. It was immediately clear, however, that the synergy of 5-HTP with hypericin was so great that the effect of 5-HTP was doubled when just a small amount of hypericin was included. They knew they had a real winner on their hands even before the market responded. What had been created by combining 5-HTP, vitamin B6 and hypericin was a product that was truly greater than the sum of the parts.

References
1. Lavie G, Valentine F, Levin B, Mazur Y, Gallo G, Lavie D, Weiner D, Meruelo D. Studies of the mechanisms of action of the antiretroviral agents hypericin and pseudohypericin. *Proc Natl Acad Sci.* 1989;,86:5963-5967.
2. Tammaro F, Xepapadakis G. Plants used in phytotherapy, cosmetics and dyeing in the Pramanda district (Epirus, North-West Greece). *J Ethnopharmacol.* 1986;16:167-174.
3. Zaichikova SG, Grinkevich NI, Barabanov EI, et al. Healing properties and determination of the upper parameters of toxicity of Hypericum herb. *Farmatsiya.* 1985;34:62-64.
4. Barbagallo C, Chisari G. Antimicrobial activity of three hypericum species. *Fitoterapia.* 1987;58:175-180.
5. Razinkov SP, Yerofeyeva LN, Khovrina MP, Lazarev AI. Validation of the use of Hypericum perforatum medicamentous form with a prolonged action to treat patients with maxillary sinusitis. *Zh Ushn Nos Gorl Bolezn.* 1989;49:43-46.
6. Martinez B, Kasper S, Ruhrmann S, Moller H-J. Hypericum in the treatment

of seasonal affective disorders. *Nervenheilkunde.* 1993;12:302-307.
7. Kubin A, Alth G, Jindra R, Jessner G, Ebermann R. Wavelength-dependent photoresponse of biological and aqueous model systems using the photodynamic plant pigment hypericin. *J Photochem Photobiol.* 1996;36:103-108.
8. Hudson J.B, Harris L, Towers GHN. The importance of light in the anti-HIV effect of hypericin. *Antiviral Res.* 1993;20:173-178.
9. De Smet PA, Nolen WA. St. John's wort as an antidepressant. *Brit Med J.* 1996;313:241-247. Editorial.
10. Linde K, Ramirez G, Mulrow CD, Pauls A, Weidenhammer W, Melchart D. St John's wort for depression: An overview and meta-analysis of randomized clinical trials. *Brit Med J.* 1996;313:253-258
11. Schmidt U, Sommer H. Extract of St. John's wort in the treatment of depression: Attention and reaction remain unimpaired. *Fortschr Med.* 1993;111:37-40.
12. Bladt S, Wagner H. Inhibition of MAO by fractions and constituents of hypericum extract. *J Geriatr Psych Neurol.* 1994;7(Suppl):S57-S59.
13. Cott J. Natural product formulations available in Europe for psychotropic indications. *Psychopharmacol Bull.* 1995;31:745-751.
14. Okpanyi SN, Weischer ML. Animal experiments on the psychotropic action of a Hypericum extract. *Arzneimit.* 1987;37:10-13.
15. Melzer R, Fricke U, Holzl J. Vasoactive properties of procyanidins from Hypericum perforatum L. in isolated porcine coronary arteries. *Arzneimit.* 1991;41:481-483.

CHAPTER 12
Meeting Your Health Goals

When first embarking upon their journey to longevity, and then repeatedly along the way as their needs change or as more options become available, serious life enhancers ask the basic question: "What should I be taking to help me live longer and feel better?"

Each month *Life Enhancement* magazine \works to help readers answer this question for themselves by presenting the most up-to-date research on products that we believe can improve your quality of life and extend your stay on this planet. But let's face it, even for those of us who have the resources and actually try to keep up with the rapidly accumulating scientific literature, the task of figuring out which products to use when and for which purpose is becoming more and more overwhelming.

In the old days you took vitamin C to prevent colds (and in the really olden days, to prevent scurvy!), vitamin E to keep your skin healthy, and maybe some calcium for strong bones and teeth. Today, though, we know that C and E at doses far above the government-mandated RDAs (ridiculously low dietary allowances!) can have a lot more uses than those listed above. And while you may need calcium to build strong bones and teeth, it works much better in the presence of hormones like estrogen and progesterone.

We also know that many more nutrient, antioxidant, and hormone supplements can be more beneficial than we previously thought, and that they all serve more than one function. In addition, for any given health goal, combining different substances can often be helpful. To complicate matters even further, certain nutrients work better in the presence of other nutrient cofactors.

We thought we'd try to cut through this confusion at least a little bit by taking a goal-oriented approach to selecting among all of the currently available supplements.

Want to improve your memory? You should be thinking about hormones like pregnenolone and DHEA and supplements like phosphatidylserine, acetyl-L-carnitine, choline, vitamins B_5 and B_6, 5-HTP and others.

Concerned about diabetes? You can focus your supplement program on helping to regulate blood sugar and improve circulation through the use of safe, effective, and natural treatments like lipoic acid, EDTA, ginkgo biloba, and IHN (inositol hexanicotinate).

Most people have more than one health goal and usually find themselves combining nutrients from different categories and discarding the duplicates. For instance, everyone can benefit from taking antiaging superhormones, but only some people would be interested in using saw palmetto for improved hair structure or prostate function.

The following tables on page 81 are representative and suggestive of how 5-HTP and related supplements can fit into your health goal program.

SLEEP

5-HTP Formulation
- Contains 5-HTP + St. John's wort (hypericin) + other cofactors
- Increases serotonin in the brain and helps trigger sleep

Take 50 to 100 mg before bed time

5-HTP
- Increases serotonin in the brain and helps trigger sleep

Take 50 to 200 mg before bedtime

Melatonin
- Restores normal sleep pattern
- Helps induce sleep
- See Superhormones for Anti-Aging for many other benefits

Take 0.5-3 mg before bedtime.

DEPRESSION AND ANXIETY

5-HTP Formulation
- Contains 5-HTP + St. John's wort (hypericin)
- Increases levels of serotonin, an important neurotransmitter, thus reducing depression and anxiety

5-HTP
- Increases levels of serotonin, an important neurotransmitter, thus reducing depression and anxiety

Pregnenolone
- Acts as a natural mood enhancer

DHEA
- Acts as a natural mood enhancer

St. John's wort
- Herb used since antiquity. Outsells Prozac® in Germany by 20 to 1.

Recommended Reading
- *Life Enhancment's 5-HTP Archives,* Valentine and Block

IMMUNE FUNCTION

Pregnenolone
- Has been shown in some studies to be helpful in lupus and fibromyalgia

DHEA
- Has been shown in some studies to be helpful in lupus and fibromyalgia

5-HTP
- Has been shown in some studies to be helpful in fibromyalgia and may also help in lupus

CHAPTER 13

5-HTP and Ephedra

INCREASED SEROTONIN LEVELS AND
THERMOGENESIS EQUAL REMARKABLE FAT LOSS

Fen-phen and Redux® (dexfenfluramine) have achieved weight-loss success, because they reduce appetite and, to a lesser degree, enhance fat-burning or thermogenesis. The probable mechanisms involved are thought to be that they elevate serotonin (5-HT) levels and stimulate adrenergic receptors. With fen-phen, each of the two drugs (fenfluramine and phentermine) worked only moderately well when used alone, but when used together the weight-loss results were significant. Apparently, there is a powerful synergetic effect when you stimulate both systems at the same time, but unfortunately, these drugs have unacceptable and serious side effects.

Fortunately, there are better — and more natural — ways to accomplish these goals than taking the dangerous fen-phen or Redux drugs. Formulations which combine 5-HTP along with ephedra and possibly white willow bark and caffeine, all of which effectively stimulate the crucial systemic functions and mechanisms (serotonergic, adrenergic, and thermogenic) can help reduce body fat, and do so safely and naturally.

5-HTP Helps Increase Serotonin,
A Natural Appetite Suppressor

As evidenced by the growing use of SSRI drugs like Prozac for weight loss, increasing serotonin levels can put a damper on appetite.

According to one British researcher, of the many appetite suppressants found to be "active" in laboratory animals, very few have clinical potential. Among the most promising candidates, he argues, are those like 5-HTP that increase the brain's levels of serotonin.[1] Others have reported that 5-HTP does not significantly increase levels elsewhere in the body.[2] A group of Italian researchers reported that 20 obese patients taking 5-HTP (900 mg/day) lost a significant amount of weight, had less carbohydrate intake, and consistently became sated earlier than a similar group taking a placebo. They concluded that since 5-HTP was well-tolerated, it could be safely used to treat obesity.[3]

Ephedra Helps Stimulate Thermogenic Function

Reducing caloric intake is just one side of the weight-loss equation. It also helps if you can burn off fat at a faster rate. Both phentermine and dexfenfluramine increase thermogenesis to a relatively small degree. **Ephedra,** on the other hand, is a more effective and safer way both to positively influence bodily function in ways that help reduce appetite[3] and help stimulate adipose brown fat cells to increase the oxidation of white fat.[5-7]

White Willow and Caffeine

Finally, there are **white willow bark** and **caffeine,** the active components of which have been shown to potentiate the function of the active ingredient in ephedra by helping to release and increase sensitivity to this primary thermogenic agent. White willow's active component and caffeine actually exert a supra-additive synergism on thermogenesis.[8-9] Moreover, the ephedra/caffeine combination simultaneously helps increase lean body tissue and promotes fat loss and preserves fat-free mass, which may contribute to its lasting effect on energy balance.[10] The combination of ephedra, the active component of white willow, and caffeine were found to be safe as well as functionally effective,[11] and with continued use even escalate thermogenesis while the effect on energy expenditure persists. There is also possibly a separate effect which helps to lower cholesterol levels.[12]

Who Would Want Fen-Phen or Redux?

Many people feel upset that fen-phen and Redux are no longer available to help them lose weight. They needn't be. Formulations which combine 5-HTP along with ephedra and possibly white willow bark and caffeine, offer all the weight loss benefits of these drugs — and more — with far fewer risks.

References

1. Blundell J. Pharmacological approaches to appetite suppression. *Trends Pharmacol.* 1991;12:147-157.
2. T. Li Kam Wa, et al. Blood and urine 5-hydroxytryptamine [serotonin] levels after administration of two 5-hydroxytryptophan precursors in normal man. *Bri J Clin Pharmacol.* 1995;39:327-329.
3. Cangiano C, Ceci F, Cascino A, et al. Eating behavior and adherence to dietary prescriptions in obese subjects treated with 5-hydroxytryptophan. *Am J Clin Nutr.* 1992;56:863-868.
4. Zarrindast M, Hosseini-Nia T, Farnoodi F. Anorectic effect of ephedrine. *Gen Pharmac.* 1987;18:559-561.
5. Pasquali R, Cesari M, Melchionda N, Steanini C, Raitano A, Labo G. Does ephedrine promote weight loss in low-energy-adapted obese women? *Int J Obesity.* 1987;11:163-168.
6. Pasquali R, Cesari M, Besteghi L, Melchionda N, Balestra V. Thermogenic agents in the treatment of human obesity: preliminary results. *Int J Obesity:*23-26.
7. Astrup A, Lundsgaard C, Madsen J, Christiensen N. Enhanced thermogenic responsiveness during chronic ephedrine treatment in man. *J Clin Nutrition.* 1985;42:83-94.
8. Astrup A, Toubro S. Thermogenic, metabolic, and cardiovascular responses to ephedrine and caffeine in man. *Int J Obes Relat Metab Disord* 1993;17 Suppl 1:S41-S43.
9. Dulloo AG, Miller DS. Ephedrine, caffeine and aspirin: "over-the-counter" drugs that interact to stimulate thermogenesis in the obese. *Nutrition.* 1989;5(1):7-9.
10. Astrup A, Toubro S, Christensen NJ, Quaade F. Pharmacology of thermogenic drugs. *Am J Clin Nutr.* 1992;55(1 Suppl):246S-248S.
11. Daly PA, Krieger DR, Dulloo AG, Young JB, Landsberg L. Ephedrine, caffeine and aspirin: safety and efficacy for treatment of human obesity. *Int J Obes Relat Metab Disord* 1993;17 Suppl 1:S73-S78.
12. Buemann B, Marckmann P, Christensen NJ, Astrup A. The effect of ephedrine plus caffeine on plasma lipids and lipoproteins during a 4.2 MJ/day diet. *Int J Obes Relat Metab Disord.* 1994;18:329-332.

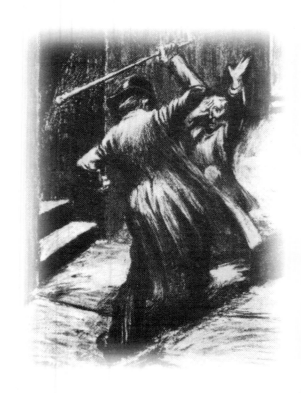

CHAPTER 14

Reducing Aggression and Violence:

The Serotonin Connection

Robert Louis Stevenson's *The Strange Case of Dr. Jekyll and Mr. Hyde* has long been viewed as a dissection of the Good and Evil that can exist within a single human being. As the well-known story goes, Jekyll ingests his formula and is temporarily transformed from a conservative, well-respected English physician into a vain, uninhibited, terrifyingly violent criminal. Not only has *Jekyll and Hyde* stood the test of time as a morality tale, studies in brain chemistry and behavior more than a century later have shown Stevenson to have had remarkable prescience regarding the role of the neurotransmitter serotonin.

Of course, Jekyll's formula was simply a fictional plot device. Other than somehow releasing some of man's baser instincts, Stevenson could have had no idea what was actually going on neurochemically.

But the 100+ years of research on brain chemistry since Stevenson wrote his Victorian classic have revealed that anything that interferes with the actions of serotonin in the brain can bring about a syndrome that resembles Jekyll's transformation to Hyde. While certainly less dramatic than the transformation described by Stevenson, serotonin deficiency bears a striking resemblance in various manifestations as an increased tendency toward anxiety, depression, out-of-control disinhibition, and violence. Conversely, enhancing the activity of the serotonin system may have exactly the opposite effects in many people. Given our current knowledge of neurochemistry, there can be little doubt that if Stevenson were writing today, Jekyll's transforming formula would have been a potent anti-serotonergic agent.

Dr. Jekyll was initially trying to prove a philosophical point when he took this potion. It's hard to imagine anyone today knowingly taking such a potion, and yet, millions of people do things every day — many of them loudly and frequently endorsed by the general medical community, the Food and Drug Administration (FDA), and many other "experts" — that significantly reduce the brain's serotonergic function. The consequences of their behavior, including increased risk of depression, anxiety, alcoholism, suicide, and violent death, are only now coming to be recognized.

Among the best studied of these Jekyll-and-Hyde-like "potions" are the cholesterol-lowering drugs (e.g., Lopid, Questran, Lescol, Mevacor, Zocor, Pravachol) and the appetite-suppressors fenfluramine (the "fen" of fen-phen fame) and dexfenfluramine (the best-selling Redux). Fenfluramine (trade names, Pondimin and Ionamin) and Redux both act by *depleting* serotonin and may permanently destroy serotonergic neurons in the brain. Even weight-loss diets that are extremely low in fat have also been noted to cause Hyde-like behavior patterns in some people. Mortality associated with violence (suicides and injuries) has been observed to increase following the use of cholesterol-lowering drugs.[1] In another study, patients with low cholesterol showed hypersensitivity to detecting anger and sadness in themselves.[2] Apparently, these too result in reduced serotonin, although usually without the permanent damage caused by fenfluramine and Redux. Both of these drugs have recently been removed from the market, in part, because of their potent anti-serotonergic effects.

Serotonin, or 5-hydroxytryptamine (5-HT), was first isolated from blood exactly 50 years ago and was later identified as a neurotransmitter in the central nervous system (CNS). As a neurotransmitter, serotonin possesses a range of effects unmatched by any similar substance. Like its catecholamine cousins, adrenalin, noradrenaline, and dopamine, serotonin acts all over the body:[3]

- In the central nervous system (CNS), 5-HT has widespread and often profound implications, including a role in sleep, appetite, memory, learning, temperature regulation, mood, sexual behavior, cardiovascular function, muscle contraction, endocrine regulation, and, of course, depression.

- Low levels of serotonin in the brain have been associated with an increased susceptibility to impulsive behavior, aggression, overeating, depression, alcohol abuse, and violent suicide. Moreover, all these behaviors seem to be linked, so that the presence of one markedly increases the risk for any of the others.

- In the blood vessels, 5-HT constricts large arteries, thus helping to balance excessive dilation required for proper normal blood pressure control.

- In the intestines, 5-HT controls GI motility (movements of the stomach and intestinal musculature).

- In the periphery, 5-HT is a major factor in platelet homeostasis which could be of benefit in the treatment of diabetes.

- As Stevenson portrayed so well in *Jekyll and Hyde,* altering serotonergic activity may even be capable of inducing profound changes in personality. In his best-selling book, *Listening to Prozac,*[4] psychiatrist Peter D. Kramer, MD, has argued that taking Prozac — or similar agents that enhance serotonergic activity — may actually help some people reconfigure their personality. This has opened a broad new avenue of use by people with no obvious psychiatric illness, who just want to feel more confident, popular, mentally nimble, and emotionally resilient.

Nerve cells synthesize 5-HT by a two-step process that begins with the essential amino acid tryptophan, which must come from dietary sources. Once taken up into a nerve cell, tryptophan is converted into 5-hydroxytryptophan (5-HTP) with the help of the enzyme tryptophan hydroxylase (TPH). 5-HTP is converted in turn to 5-HT (serotonin). Studies show that taking supplements of tryptophan or 5-HTP will increase the amount of serotonin available for use by neurons.[5] (Note: Chronic stress, with its concomitant increases in cortisol, can inhibit the conversion of dietary tryptophan to 5-HTP, but not 5-HTP to 5-HT. This suggests an advantage of using 5-HTP instead of tryptophan for relieving problems associated with stress.)

The first hints that serotonin played an important role in regulating aggressive behaviors came in the mid-1970s when researchers doing postmortem examinations on suicide victims noticed that these people had reduced levels of a major metabolite of serotonin called 5-hydroxyindoleacetic acid (5-HIAA) in their cerebrospinal fluid (CSF).[6] Subsequent studies found lower levels of 5-HIAA in people who had attempted suicide, had severe depression, or had shown tendencies to harm themselves or others.[7]

Cross-Species Aggression Control
Serotonin's influence over aggressive tendencies goes way back in the evolution of life. Studies over a wide range of species, from crustaceans to fish to lizards to hamsters to mice to dogs to nonhuman primates to human beings, have all demonstrated essentially the same results: reducing serotonergic activity leads to increases in aggressive behavior, and enhancing serotonergic function decreases aggressive behavior.[7-13]

This relationship can have some interesting ramifications. For example, animals that have been selected for domesticity (i.e., reduced aggression) may have higher brain levels of serotonin than their wild counterparts.

Russian researchers studying silver foxes, for example, found that those selected for more than 30 years for tame behavior and no defensive reactions to humans had higher levels of both serotonin and 5-HIAA in various regions of the brain, compared with wild silver foxes bred in captivity. They also found higher levels of tryptophan hydroxylase (TPH, the primary enzyme involved in the production of serotonin) and lower levels of monoamine oxidase (MAO, the enzyme that removes serotonin from the synapse) in the domesticated animals.[14]

So sensitive is this serotonergic system that natural variations in serotonin levels among animals on a normal diet can affect their behavior in profound ways, possibly even spelling the difference between life and death. A team of researchers from the National Institute of Alcohol Abuse and Alcoholism (NIAAA) has been studying a colony of free-ranging rhesus monkeys living on a

475-acre sea island. Among their most important findings: those monkeys with the lowest CSF levels of 5-HIAA (indicating low serotonin) stand the greatest chance of getting injured and/or dying young.[15]

The NIAAA researchers first took blood and CSF samples from 49 2-year-old male rhesus monkeys and then set them free on the island. Over the next 4 years, they closely and systematically observed the animals' behavior, paying particular attention to aggressive interactions. At the end of 4 years, six of the monkeys were dead, and five others were missing and presumed dead.

In retrospect, the animals' fate could have been predicted by their CSF 5-HIAA at age 2. Not a single monkey from the highest CSF 5-HIAA concentration quartile died or went missing. By contrast, 46% of the dead or missing came from the low end of the 5-HIAA concentration spectrum, with all but one coming from the two bottom quartiles.

The authors also observed that the monkeys that turned up dead or missing were the ones most likely to initiate or escalate aggressive encounters. Not surprisingly, these aggressive animals stood the greatest risk of suffering trauma or injury. Of the six animals whose death could be ascertained, four had died as a result of injuries sustained in a fight, and all four had had among the lowest levels of 5-HIAA at age 2.

More subtle variations in social behavior have also been related to serotonin levels.[16] Among 26 adolescent male rhesus monkeys from the same island colony, for example, those with the highest levels of CSF 5-HIAA concentration were seen spending more time grooming other group members and staying in close proximity to others. Those with the lowest levels of CSF 5-HIAA were more likely to leave their social groups at a younger age, an indication of lower social competence. Low CSF 5-HIAA animals were also observed to take greater physical risks, including longer leaps in the trees at greater heights. The authors suggested that this behavior indicated impaired impulse control.[15]

The drug parachlorophenylalanine (pCPA) inhibits serotonin synthesis, reducing the availability of serotonin in the brain. When pCPA is given to vervet monkeys, it makes them irritable and aggressive. When these same animals are then treated with the selective serotonin reuptake inhibitor (SSRI) Prozac or the serotonin precursor 5-hydroxytryptophan (5-HTP), both of which increase the availability of serotonin in brain synapses, there is no increase in aggressiveness.[16]

Since the body normally synthesizes serotonin from dietary tryptophan, altering the diet can also change behavior. For example, animals placed on a tryptophan-free diet, leading to reduced serotonin levels, have greater aggressive tendencies, especially during competitive social interactions like feeding.[16]

When it comes to the need for serotonin, human beings appear to be no different than their cousins in the swamp. Feed us too little tryptophan and we can become impulsive, depressive, aggressive, and violent. Feed us enough tryptophan or 5-HTP and these traits diminish or disappear.

In one study, human subjects ingested an amino acid beverage that was devoid of tryptophan. This "unbalanced" mixture not only deprives the body of new tryptophan for making serotonin, it also interferes with the body's utilization of the tryptophan already in the brain. Within 5 or 6 hours after taking this formulation, subjects were found to have an 80% or more drop in plasma tryptophan levels and a concomitant "lowering" of mood.[19]

Researchers at the University of Texas, Houston Health Science Center gave this low-tryptophan formula (25 gm or 100 gm) to 10 healthy men in a controlled laboratory setting following a 24-hr low-tryptophan diet. They then observed the men's behavior and noted any aggressive tendencies. The men taking the 100-gm formula (lower tryptophan) showed a significant increase in aggressive responding (compared with baseline) within only 5 hours. The 25-gm formula took 6 hours to produce the same effect.[20]

Violence: Inner- and Outer-Directed
Researchers have found that violence related to low serotonin can be either inner- or outer-directed. A group of Danish scientists measured 5-HIAA and other serotonin metabolites in the CSF of 16 men convicted of criminal homicide, 22 men who attempted suicide and 39 healthy male controls. The lowest levels of 5-HIAA

were found in those men who had killed a sexual partner or had attempted suicide.[21]

Investigators at Columbia University evaluated personality variables and CSF 5-HIAA levels in 26 patients considered to be "self-mutilators."[22] In addition to serotonergic dysfunction indicated by lower 5-HIAA levels, compared with controls, self-mutilators were found to have significantly more severe character pathology and greater lifetime aggression; they were more antisocial, and had greater impulsivity, chronic anger, and somatic anxiety.

Suicide, the ultimate expression of "auto-aggression," has long been linked to low serotonin levels. In one meta-analysis, five out of seven studies reported reduced levels of serotonin and/or 5-HIAA in the brain stems of suicide victims. Reduced brain levels were also seen in those who had attempted suicide but failed.[23]

As one might expect, drugs that interfere with serotonergic function can increase aggressive behavior. British scientists gave 35 healthy subjects dexfenfluramine (better known as the recently departed diet drug Redux), which is known to deplete serotonin (sometimes permanently). Using a questionnaire to assess the subjects' hostility and aggression, they found that dexfenfluramine treatment in male subjects (but not females) was associated with an increase in hostility and aggression scores.[23]

Cholesterol and Violent Death

One of the more puzzling findings of recent years has been an increase in depression, suicide and violent death among people taking cholesterol-lowering drugs or on severely cholesterol-restricted diets.[24-29] In other words, taking these widely recommended steps to reduce your risk of death from coronary heart disease and stroke may place you at greater risk of serious depression, suicide, or death due to violence.

How can this be? Although the exact relationships have yet to be worked out, it appears that the missing link between low cholesterol and violent death may be serotonin. This association was demonstrated most clearly in a study of juvenile cynomolgus monkeys fed a diet high in fat and either high or low in cholesterol. The animals were then observed for 8 months.

The researchers found that animals on the low-cholesterol diet were more aggressive, less affiliative, and had significantly lower CSF 5-HIAA levels compared with those on the high-cholesterol diet. "These monkeys went at it hammer and tong," says Jay Kaplan, PhD, who led the study. "They engaged in more contact aggression — highly charged impulsive fighting — than the other monkeys.[30] Kaplan believes that people on low-cholesterol diets may be experiencing the same kind of impulsive aggression.

Kaplan raises the heretical question, "Can low-fat, low-cholesterol diets actually do some people more harm than good?" "For people who already have low serotonergic activity, a low-cholesterol diet might shove them across some threshold that makes them more likely to do things they might not otherwise do," he said.[31]

The precise mechanism linking cholesterol, serotonin, and aggressive behavior has yet to be elaborated, although a few hypotheses have been put forward. One hypothesis emphasizes cholesterol's role as a major component of brain cell membranes. Reducing cholesterol to too low a level may affect the fluidity and viscosity of these membranes, which contain the receptors for serotonin.[29]

According to another hypothesis, low cholesterol may be accompanied by a decrease in serum-free tryptophan, which results in a decrease in serotonin synthesis. To test this hypothesis, a group of Dutch researchers compared serotonin metabolism in subjects whose serum cholesterol was chronically low with another group whose cholesterol levels were normal. They found that plasma serotonin levels were 21.3% lower in the low-cholesterol group, suggesting a disruption of serotonin metabolism.[32]

Serotonin, Alcohol & Aggression

The relationship between alcohol, depression, and violence is well-known. A high proportion of suicide victims are found to have been drinking heavily at the time of their death. Similarly, perpetrators (and victims!) of violent crimes are often intoxicated at the time of the crime.[33]

In animal studies, some drugs that decrease serotonin activity increase alcohol consumption. But when animals are given serotonin, tryptophan, 5-HTP, or an SSRI, their alcohol consumption drops. Rats that have been bred to prefer drinking alcohol to water have been found to have reduced serotonin activity compared with normal rats.[34]

Human studies have consistently demonstrated reduced alcohol intake among various groups, including social drinkers and alcohol-dependent males, taking SSRIs.[34] Alcoholics have also been shown to have reduced serotonin function activity as indicated by low levels of 5-HIAA.[35, 36]

Chronic alcohol use actually appears to increase serotonin concentration in the CSF and to facilitate serotonin activity. However, as soon as drinking stops, serotonin levels drop concurrently with the appearance of alcohol withdrawal symptoms. It is thought that the decrease in serotonin associated with withdrawal may contribute to the craving for alcohol that occurs during this period. If abstinence is maintained, serotonin levels gradually return to normal.[34]

(This seems to suggest that, if you're going to have a drink, take a 5-HTP capsule with it, or in advance, or on a regular basis. Although informal studies have been done to test this hypothesis, you may find yourself less likely to want a second (or third) drink. And you might have fewer withdrawal symptoms and hangovers.)

There's little doubt, though, that low serotonin activity combined with high alcohol intake is a dangerous combination. Finnish researchers have found that brain serotonin turnover is low among alcoholic, impulsive, habitually violent offenders. Not only does low serotonin seem to predispose people to alcoholism, it may also make them more aggressive, violent, and suicidal. The risk of violence or other antisocial behavior may be compounded in men whose testosterone levels are high.[37, 38]

How does serotonin modulate these responses? Researchers Robert O. Pihl and colleagues at McGill University speculate that serotonin modifies the response to threat. In people with normal serotonin function, anxiety (the emotional response to threat) inhibits socially inappropriate responses, such as aggression. In people with depleted serotonin, however, anxiety loses its inhibitory effect while retaining its emotional intensity. As a result of this imbalance, a person might become aggressive despite the intense anxiety induced by the threat of punishment.[34]

Pihl et al state that people with low serotonin are likely "to appear depressed and aggressive, more driven by appetites (more motivated by food, water, sex, and drugs of abuse), and more impulsive (less able to control behavior) in the face of threat." They may also be more likely to use aggression to achieve rewards or deter punishment, and they may be less sensitive to social control of such behavior. Specifically with regard to alcohol, decreased serotonin may lead to an inability to terminate drinking once started. And if a person with low serotonin starts drinking, the result is likely to be an increase in aggressive behavior. "The combination of impulsivity [due to low serotonin] with alcohol-induced fearlessness and hyperactivity appears prone to produce aggressive acts or to culminate in victimization," the authors write.[34]

Reversing Serotonin Deficiency

If low serotonergic function can lead to aggressive and violent behavior, can reversing a serotonin deficiency restore more normal behavior? Although this area has not been studied systematically, some evidence suggests that it may. Serotonergic function can be enhanced in two basic ways: by providing the metabolic precursors for serotonin or by preventing the inactivation of serotonin that is released into the synapse.

Increasing serotonin synthesis. When taken up into neurons, the amino acids tryptophan and 5-HTP are converted into serotonin. Most studies with these amino acid precursors have involved people with depression, but the results are encouraging, particularly for 5-HTP. In one double-blind study, 5-HTP was found to be equal to an SSRI antidepressant drug in alleviating depression with fewer and less severe adverse effects. In addition to alleviating depression, 5-HTP seems to be capable of alleviating a wide range of symptoms of what Pöldinger has called the "serotonin deficiency syndrome," which includes depression, anxiety, aggression, sleep disturbances, obsessive-compulsive traits, and other behavioral manifestations.[5]

In another double-blind study, researchers gave tryptophan or placebo to a group of aggressive psychiatric inpatients. Injections of antipsychotics and other medications were also given, as needed, to control violent behavior. Although tryptophan treatment had no effect on the number of violent incidents, it significantly reduced the need for injections of antipsychotic and sedative drugs.[39]

Inhibiting serotonin inactivation. Serotonin released into the synaptic cleft is normally inactivated by either being taken back up into the neuron that released it (reuptake) or metabolized by the enzyme monoamine oxidase (MAO). Drugs that inhibit this inactivation, including the selective serotonin reuptake inhibitors (SSRIs) like Prozac (fluoxetine) and others and, to a lesser degree, MAO inhibitors, have been shown to be effective antidepressants.

A few studies suggest that SSRIs may also be able to control aggressive or violent behavior. In one study in dogs, for example, fluoxetine was found to be effective in managing dominance aggression.[40] In humans, preliminary data suggest that fluoxetine may also decrease aggressive behavior and feelings of anger or hostility.[41] In adult male lizards (Anolis carolinensis), fluoxetine injections significantly reduced aggressive responding in males.[12]

Toward a Better World

Dr. Jekyll's formula dramatically exposed mankind's darker side. With the benefit of a century of neurobiological research, we can only marvel at Stevenson's insights, not only into the human character, but also into its biochemical basis. While he in all likelihood had no concept of serotonergic mechanisms, he described with astonishing accuracy the behavioral effects of serotonin depletion.

It's probably safe to say that the world would be a better, safer, happier place if everyone's serotonergic functioning could be maintained at optimal levels. Scientific evidence confirms that preventing or restoring serotonin depletion results in decreased depression, alcoholism, aggression, violence, appetite disorders, sleeping disorders, migraine headaches, and many other benefits. While this is not to say that tryptophan or 5-HTP should be added to the drinking water, the growing body of literature on the adverse effects of reduced serotonin function, including those caused by medically sanctioned practices such as following a low-cholesterol diet, taking cholesterol-reducing drugs or serotonin-depleting drugs (e.g., fenfluramine and Redux) should turn our thoughts to serious consideration of the benefits of precursor dietary supplementation. The proven and potential benefits of enhancing serotonergic function, especially by taking serotonin precursors such as 5-HTP or tryptophan [should the latter ever become available again] are enough to allow us to visualize the day when the Hydes are permanently disabled and the good Dr. Jekylls are empowered.

References

1. Penttinen J. Hypothesis: low serum cholesterol, suicide, and interleukin-2. *Am J Epidemiol.* 1995;141:716-718.
2. Guggenheim CB, Foster HG Jr.Serum cholesterol and perception of anger and sadness. *Psychol Rep.* 1995;77:1343-1345.
3. Borne R. Serotonin: The Neurotransmitter for the '90s. *Drug Topics.* 1994;October 10:108.
4. Kramer P. *Listening to Prozac.* New York: Viking; 1993.
5. Pöldinger W, Calanchini B, Schwarz W. A functional-dimensional approach to depression: serotonin deficiency as a target syndrome in a comparison of 5-hydroxytryptophan and fluvoxamine. *Psychopathology.* 1991;24:53-81.
6. Lloyd K, Farley L, Deck J, Horykiewicz O. Serotonin and 5-hydroxy-indoleacetic acid in discrete areas of the brainstem of suicide victims and control patients. *Adv Biochem Psychopharm.* 1974;11:387-398.
7. Huber R, Smith K, Delago A, Isaksson K, Krvitz E. Serotonin and aggressive motivation in crustaceans: altering the decision to retreat. *Proc Natl Acad Sci.* 1997;94:5939-5942.
8. Adams C, Liley N, Gorzalka B. PCPA increases aggression in male firemouth cichlids. *Pharmacology.* 1996;53:328-330.
9. Ferris C, Melloni Jr R, Koppel G, Perry K, Fuller R, Delville Y. Vasopressin/serotonin interactions in the anterior hypothalamus control aggressive behavior in golden hamsters. *Neurosci.* 1997;17:4331-4340.
10. Amstislavskaya T, Kudryavtseva N. Effect of repeated experience of victory and defeat in daily agonistic confrontations on brain tryptophan hydroxylase activity. *FEBS Lett.* 1997;406:106-108.
11. Reisner I, Mann J, Stanley M, Huang Y, Houpt K. Comparison of cerebrospinal fluid monoamine metabolite levels in dominant-aggressive

and non-aggressive dogs. *Brain Res.* 1996;714:57-64.

12. Deckel A. Behavioral changes in Anolis carolinensis following injection with fluoxetine. *Behav Brain Res.* 1996;78:175-182.

13. Higley J, Suomi S, Linnoila M. A nonhuman primate model of type II alcoholism? Part 2. Diminished social competence and excessive aggression correlates with low cerebrospinal fluid 5-hydroxyindoleacetic acid concentrations. *Alcohol Clin Exp Res.* 1996;20:643-650.

14. Popova N, Voitenko N, Kulikov A, Avgustinovich D. Evidence for the involvement of central serotonin in mechanism of domestication of silver foxes. *Pharmacol Biochem Behav.* 1991;40:751-756.

15. Higley J, Mehlman P, Higley S, et al. Excessive mortality in young free-ranging male nonhuman primates with low cerebrospinal fluid 5-hydroxyindoleacetic acid concentrations. *Arch Gen Psychiatry.* 1996;53:537-543.

16. Mehlman P, Higley J, Faucher I, et al. Correlation of CSF 5-HIAA concentration with sociality and the timing of emigration in free-ranging primates. *Am J Psychiatry.* 1995;152:907-913.

17. Mehlman P, Higley J, Faucher I, et al. Low CSF-HIAA concentrations and severe aggression and impaired impulse control in nonhuman primates. *Am J Psychiatry.* 1995;151:1485-1491.

18. Chamberlain B, Ervin F, Pihl R, Young S. The effect of raising or lowering tryptophan levels on aggression in vervet monkeys. *Pharmacol Biochem Behav.* 1987;28:503-510.

19. Young S, Tourjman S, Teff K, Pihl R, Anderson G. The effect of lowering plasma tryptophan on food selection in normal males. *Pharmacol Biochem Behav.* 1988;31:149-152.

20. Collins D, Davis C, Cherek D. Tryptophan depletion and aggressive responding in healthy males. *Psychopharmacology.* 1996;126:97-103.

21. Lidberg L, Tuck J, Asberg M, Scalia-Tomba G, Bertilsson L. Homicide, suicide and CSF 5-HIAA. *Acta Psychiatr Scand.* 1985;71:230-236.

22. Simeon D, Stanley B, Frances A, Mann J, Winchel R, Stanley M. Self-mutilation in personality disorders: psychological and biological correlates. *Am J Psychiatry.* 1992;149:221-226.

23. Mann J, Arango V, Underwood M. Serotonin and suicidal behavior. *Ann NY Acad Sci.* 1990;600:476-484.

24. Cleare A, Bond A. Does central serotonergic function correlate inversely with aggression? A study using D-fenfluramine in healthy subjects. *Psychiatry Res.* 1997;69:89-95.

25. Renzo R, Bertozzi B, Barbisoni P, Trabucchi M. Risk of depression is higher in elderly patients with lowest serum chholesterol values (letter). *Br Med J.* 1996;312:1296-1299.

26. Kunugi H, Takei N, Aoki H, Nanko S. Low serum cholesterol in suicide attempters. *Biol Psychiatry.* 1997;41:196-200.

27. Rybakowski J, Ainiyet J, Szajnerman Z, Zakrzewska M. The study of the relationship between cholesterol and lipid concentration and suicidal behavior in patients with schizophrenia affective illness. *Psychiatr Pol.* 1996;30:699-712.

28. Santiago J, Dalen J. Cholesterol and violent behavior. *Arch Intern Med.*

1994;154:1317-1321.

29. Hawthon K, Cowen P, Owens D, Bond A, Elliott M. Low serum cholesterol and suicide. *Br J Psychiatry*. 1993;162:818-825.

30. Kaplan J, Shively C, Fontenot M, et al. Demonstration of an association among dietary cholesterol, central serotonergic activity, and social behavior. *Psychosom Med*. 1994;56:479-484.

31. Anonymous. The cholesterol conundrum. *Psychology Today*. 1995;28:16.

32. Steegmans P, Fekkes D, Hoes A, Bak A, Does E, Grobbee D. Low serum cholesterol concentration and serotonin metabolism in man. *Br Med J*. 1996;312:221.

33. Murdoch D, Pihl R, Ross D. Alcohol and crimes of violence: present issues. *Int J Addict*. 1990;25:1065-1081.

34. Pihl R, Peterson J. Alcohol, serotonin and aggression. *Alcohol Health Res World*. 1993;17:113-117.

35. Banki C. Factors influencing monoamine metabolites and tryptophan in patients with alcohol dependence. *J Neural Transm*. 1981;50:89-101.

36. LeMarquand D, Pihl R, Benkelfat C. Serotonin and alcohol intake, abuse, and dependence: clinical evidence. *Biol Psychiatry*. 1994;36:326-337.

37. Virkkunen M, Goldman D, Linnoila M. Serotonin in alcoholic violent male offenders. *Ciba Foundation Symposium*. 1996;194:168-177.

38. Virkkunen M, Rawlings R, Tokola R, et al. CSF biochemistries, glucose metabolism, and diurnal activity rhythms in alcoholic, violent offenders, fire setters, and healthy volunteers. *Arch Gen Psychiatry*. 1994;51:20-27.

39. Volavka J, Crowner M, Brizer D, Convit A, Van Praag H, Suckow R. Tryptophan treatment of aggressive psychiatric inpatients. *Biol Psychiatry*. 1990;28:728-732.

40. Dodman N, Donelly R, Shuster L, Mertens P, Rand W, Miczek K. Use of fluoxetine to treat dominance aggression in dogs. *J Am Vet Assoc*. 1996;209:1585-1587.

41. Fuller R. Fluoxetine effects on serotonin function and aggressive behavior. *Ann NY Acad Sci*. 1996;794:90-97.

CHAPTER 15

Waist Size Reduction: Three Easy Ways

Despite the omnipresent emphasis in our culture on the value of physical activity and healthful, moderate eating habits, the American waistline continues to expand. Obesity and weight gain have reached epidemic proportions. Although the incidence of obesity in adults increased by only about 1% between 1960 and 1980, between 1988 and 1994, it had jumped by nearly 10% — from 15% to 25% in the general population.[1]

Concern about the growing problem of being overweight stems largely from the fact that too much body fat is a major risk factor for a large number of serious chronic diseases, including diabetes mellitus, cardiovascular disease, hyperinsulinemia, atherosclerosis, hypertension, and some types of cancer.[2,3] After tobacco use, obesity is the second leading cause of preventable death.[4]

Body Mass Index

Obesity has been defined as the excessive storage of body fat,[5] but specifying exactly what is excessive has been somewhat problematic. The current standard for assessing obesity is the **body mass index (BMI)**, which is defined as body weight (in kilograms) divided by the square of the height (in meters), or [body weight (kg)/m2].[6] Although body weight may increase as a result of muscle and adipose tissue, BMI has been shown to correlate well with both adiposity and health risks.[7]

To determine your BMI, divide your weight in kilograms by the square of your height in meters. If you are among the

Table 1. What Is Your BMI?*

Match your weight† with your height

Obesity Grade:	1	2	3	4	5	6
Definition:	Overweight	Obesity	Significant Obesity	Morbid Obesity	Super Obesity	Super-morbid Obesity
BMI:	25	30	35	40	45	50
Height:						
4'10"	120	144	167	191	215	239
4'11"	124	149	174	198	223	248
5'0"	128	153	179	205	230	256
5'1"	132	159	185	212	238	265
5'2"	137	164	191	219	246	273
5'3"	141	169	198	226	254	282
5'4"	146	175	204	233	262	291
5'5"	150	181	211	241	271	301
5'6"	155	186	217	248	279	310
5'7"	160	192	224	256	288	320
5'8"	164	197	230	263	296	329
5'9"	169	203	237	271	305	338
5'10"	174	209	244	279	313	348
5'11"	179	215	251	287	322	358
6'0"	185	222	259	295	332	369
6'1"	190	228	265	303	341	379
6'2"	195	233	272	311	350	389
6'3"	200	240	280	320	360	400
6'4"	206	247	288	329	370	411

* Weight is without shoes and clothes.
† If you have a large frame and/or a high muscle/fat ratio, this chart may place you mistakenly into a risk category.

many decimally challenged in the US, you can multiply your weight in pounds by 703; then divide by the square of your height in inches. For example, if you weigh 130 pounds and are 5'4" (64") tall, your BMI is (130 * 703)/(64 * 64) = 22.3. You can also approximate your BMI by finding your height and weight on Table 1.

According to current definitions, you are considered to be "overweight" if your BMI is greater than 25. You fall into the "obese" class if your BMI is greater than 30. Individuals with a BMI greater than 27 — which amounts to about 120% of desirable weight for your height — are considered to be at increased risk for morbidity and mortality.[7-10]

Recent studies have shown that even minimal increases in a person's BMI are associated with an increased risk of both fatal and nonfatal heart attacks, even if the person has no other risk factors for heart disease. At the same time, as little as a 5% weight loss has been shown to reduce or eliminate disorders associated with obesity.[11]

Waist-to-Hip Ratio

It's not only how much fat you're carrying around, but also how you carry it. **Fat distribution,** as measured by the **waist-to-hip ratio (WHR)** and **waist circumference,** for example, have been found to be good predictors of long-term complications.[12] Ideally in women, the waist should be narrower than the hip — the classic "hourglass" figure. The familiar "spare-tire" fat distribution, in which the waist is wider than the hip, is an indication of potential health risks. This is true for men as well, although a man's risk ratio is different from a woman's.

To find out your waist-to-hip ratio, measure the waist at its narrowest point, then measure the hips at their widest point. Divide the waist measurement by the hip measurement. For a woman with a 35" waist and 46" hips, the WHR would be: 35/46 = 0.76. Women with a waist-to-hip ratio greater than 0.8 and men with a waist-to-hip ratio greater than 1.0 are at increased health risk because of their fat distribution.

Growing Older, Growing Fatter

Vladimir Dilman, MD, PhD, one of the giants of antiaging medicine, observed that an increase in body weight is a "normal" accompaniment of advancing age.[13] Even if you don't gain body weight as you age, you may still be increasing the amount of fat relative to lean muscle and bone mass for two primary reasons:

- Fat deposits typically increase with age, while bone and muscle mass decline
- Fat cells themselves grow larger with age

Dilman believed that age-associated obesity was caused by such factors as age-related hyperglycemia and hyperinsulinemia, decreased physical activity, and excessive food intake (particularly carbohydrates). He reasoned that people tend to overeat as they age because the hypothalamic brain centers that control satiety become less sensitive to the signals provided by blood glucose levels. "Consequently, with increasing age, those whose food consumption depends on their appetite are inevitably on a path to obesity," wrote Dilman.[13]

Reducing Stored Fat

Unfortunately, as Dilman demonstrated and as most people over age 40 eventually find out for themselves, the older one gets, the harder it is to keep the fat off. To most people — including most physicians and weight-loss "experts," caloric reduction is the key to weight (fat) loss. Caloric reduction is to be accomplished by drastically cutting fat intake in favor of a diet high in carbohydrates.

The only problem with this diet is that it doesn't work. In the long run, 95% of people who lose weight primarily by caloric/fat restriction gain the lost weight back, and they gain it back mostly as fat, rather than lean muscle or bone.

Appetite Suppression + Thermogenesis:
The Better Way to Lose Fat

Although it cannot be the whole answer, caloric restriction remains an important element in any weight-loss program. But, if

THREE FAT-LOSS CHOICES

There are three formulations that should be considered when your goal is to provide fat-loss, lean tissue gain/preservation benefits of appetite suppression and enhanced thermogenesis, with none of the risks of dangerous drugs like methamphetamine, fen-phen, and Redux.

- A formulation containing **ephedra + caffeine, yohimbe, DHEA,** and **white willow** should help reduce appetite and hit body fat with a 1-2-3 thermogenic punch.

- **Another formulation involving** a slightly different tack would contain **ephedra + caffeine + white willow** to stimulate thermogenesis, and also **5-HTP** to help with appetite satisfaction. This unique combination helps enhance fat loss with less of a stimulant effect than the DHEA version above.

- **Finally, there** is the classic GH-releasing formula containing **arginine** plus cofactors **vitamin B5** and **choline** for enhanced, natural GH release. This formulation can be used with either of the two above formulations based on either DHEA and ephedra or 5-HTP and ephedra.

Dilman is right, and appetite becomes a less and less reliable clue to the number of calories the body requires, then how can we best adjust appetite to a level more in keeping with our physiologic needs?

One means that has been used repeatedly over the last 30 or 40 years has been appetite-suppressing drugs. The best known of these have been the amphetamines, fen-phen (fenfluramine/phentermine), and dexfenfluramine (Redux), which work by a combination of adrenergic and serotonergic mechanisms. Although these drugs proved to be generally effective in reducing caloric intake, they have turned out to be dangerous, causing serious or even fatal side effects at a rate that led to their recent removal from the marketplace.

A far safer avenue appears to be enhancing serotonergic function using metabolic precursors of serotonin, such as the amino acid tryptophan and the naturally derived 5-hydroxytryptophan (5-HTP). Studies have demonstrated that increasing serotonin levels can put a damper on appetite. According to one British researcher, of the many appetite suppressants found to be "active" in laboratory animals, very few have clinical potential. Among the most promising candidates, he argues, are those like 5-HTP that increase central levels of serotonin.[14] A group of Italian researchers reporting on a small study found that 20 obese patients taking 5-HTP (900 mg/day) lost a significant amount of weight, had lower carbohydrate intake, and consistently became sated earlier than a similar group taking a placebo. They concluded that since 5-HTP was well-tolerated, it could be safely used to treat obesity.[15]

Too often ignored by conventional weight-loss programs is the value of enhanced *thermogenesis.* Thermogenesis is the process by which the body uses its fat stores to provide energy for its many functions. Fat is literally burned to generate heat *(thermo* = heat, *genesis* = generation). The more fat the body uses up in this way, the less it has to store in that "spare tire." If you can "turn up the flame" on your fat stores, you'll lose weight and fat, reduce your BMI and your WHR.

The ancient Chinese herb ephedra (ma huang) has long been recognized as a safe and effective way both to reduce appetite[16]

and stimulate thermogenesis.[17-19] Furthermore, studies have shown that when ephedra is combined with substances such as caffeine, theophylline, and/or yohimbe and white willow, its thermogenic effects are amplified.[20]

The ephedra/caffeine combination simultaneously has been shown to help *increase lean body tissue and preserve fat-free mass, while promoting fat loss.* In a Danish study in obese women, the combination of ephedrine and caffeine was superior to placebo in preserving fat-free mass and enhancing fat loss. The effect was calculated to be due to appetite suppression (75%) and thermogenesis (25%).[21]

The addition of the active ingredient including white willow (which contains acetylsalicylic acid, generically known as aspirin) to ephedra/caffeine has also been found to be functionally effective in producing "modest, sustained weight loss even without prescribed caloric restriction." The authors speculated that restricting caloric intake might make this treatment even more effective. The combination was reported to be "well-tolerated in otherwise healthy obese subjects."[22]

Growth Hormone Release

Not to be overlooked in any weight-loss program is the importance of growth hormone (GH) release. Diminished secretion of growth hormone is responsible in part for the age-related decrease in lean body mass and the expansion of adipose-tissue mass.[23] Administration of recombinant GH has been shown to produce dramatic changes in body composition, including increases in lean body mass and reductions in fat mass.[24]

Growth hormone injections are out of the question for most people because of cost, the need for a prescription (recombinant hGH has not been approved by the FDA for treating obesity), and medical concerns about various side effects. However, ingesting the amino acid arginine has repeatedly been shown to result in a natural release of GH from the pituitary gland,[25] and appears to provide the same benefits of reducing fat mass and increasing lean tissue mass.

References

1. Kuczmarski R, Flegal K, Campbell S, Johnson C. Increasing prevalence of overweight among US adults. The National Health and Nutrition Examination Surveys, 1960 to 1991. *JAMA*. 1994;272:205-211.
2. Pi-Sunyer F. Medical hazards of obesity. *Ann Intern Med*. 1993;119:655-660.
3. Stunkard A. Current views on obesity. *Am J Med*. 1996;100:230-236.
4. McGinnis J, Foege W. Actual causes of death in the United States. *JAMA*. 1993;170:2207-2212.
5. Colditz G, Wolf A. The public health impact of obesity. In: Angel A, Anderson C, Bouchard D, et al, eds. *Progress in Obesity Research*. London: John Libbey & Co.; 1996:517-523.
6. NIH Technology Assessment Panel. Methods for voluntary weight loss and control. *Ann Intern Med*. 1993;119:764-770.
7. Olefsky J. *Obesity*. New York: McGraw-Hill Inc; 1994:446-452.
8. Doering P. Weight control products. *Handbook of Nonprescription Drugs*, 11th ed. Washington, DC: American Pharmaceutical Association; 1996:423-445.
9. Dwyer J. Medical evaluation and classification of obesity. In: Blackburn G, Kanders B, eds. *Obesity: Pathophysiology, Psychology, and Treatment*. New York: Chapman & Hall; 1994:9-38.
10. Wadden T. Obesity. In: Kaplan H, Saddock B, eds. *Comprehensive Textbook of Psychiatry*. Baltimore, MD: Williams and Wilkins; 1995:1481-1491.
11. Blackburn G. Effect of degree of weight loss on health benefits. *Obesity Research*. 1995;3:211-216.
12. Chan J, Rimm E, Colditz G, Stampfer M, Willett W. Obesity, fat distribution, and weight gain as risk factors for clinical diabetes in men. *Diabetes Care*. 1994;17:961-969.
13. Dilman V, Dean W. *The Neuroendocrine Theory of Aging and Degeneration*. Pensacola, FL: The Center for BioGerontology; 1992.
14. Blundell J. Pharmacological approches to appetite suppression. *Trends Pharmacol*. 1991;12:147-157.
15. Cangiano C, Ceci F, Cascino A, et al. Eating behavior and adherence to dietary prescriptions in obese subjects treated with 5-hydroxytryptophan. *Am J Clin Nutr*. 1992;56:863-868.
16. Zarrindast M, Hosseini-Nia T, Farnoodi F. Anorectic effect of ephedrine. *Gen Pharmac*. 1987;18:559-561.
17. Pasquali R, Cesari M, Besteghi L, Melchionda N, Balestra V. Thermogenic agents in the treatment of human obesity: preliminary results. *Int J Obesity*:23-26.
18. Pasquali R, Cesari M, Melchionda N, Steanini C, Raitano A, Labo G. Does ephedrine promote weight loss in low-energy-adapted obese women? *Int J Obesity*. 1987;11:163-168.
19. Astrup A, Lundsgaard C, Madsen J, Christiensen N. Enhanced thermogenic responsiveness during chronic ephedrine treatment in man. *J Clin Nutrition*. 1985;42:83-94.
20. Malchow-Møller A, Larsen S, Hey H, Stokholm K, Juhl E, Quaade F.

Ephedrine as an anorectic: the story of the "Elsinore pill". *Int J Obesity*. 1981;5:183-187.

21. Astrup A, Toubro S, Christensen N, Quaade F. Pharmacology of thermogenic drugs. *Am J Clin Nutr*. 1992;55 (1 Suppl):246S-248S.

22. Daly P, Krieger D, Dulloo A, Young J, Landsberg L. Ephedrine, caffeine and aspirin: safety and efficacy for treatment of human obesity. *Int J Obes Relat Metab Disord*. 1993;17 (Suppl 1):S73-S78.

23. Rudman D, Feller A, Nagraj H, et al. Effects of human growth hormone in men over 60 years old. *N Engl J Med*. 1990;323:1-6.

24. Carroll P, Littlewood R, Weissberger A, Bogalho P, McGauley G, Sonksen P. The effects of two doses of replacement growth hormone on the biochemical, body composition and psychological profiles of growth hormone-deficient adults. *Eur J Endocrinol*. 1997;137:146-153.

25. Koppeschaar H, ten Horn C, Thijssen J, Page M, Dieguez C. Differential effects of arginine on growth hormone releasing hormone and insulin-induced growth hormone secretion. *Clin Endocrinol*. 1992;36:487-490.

CHAPTER 16

5-HTP MAY HELP

Make Spring Come Sooner

WHAT TO DO ABOUT SEASONAL AFFECTIVE/EATING DISORDER

Have you been feeling a little tired lately? Has it been more difficult to get out of bed? Does another report of forthcoming torrential rains, blizzards, mud slides, floods, road shoreline erosion or inclement conditions seem to add to your lethargic, listless, sluggish, even depressive moods? Rest assured, you're not alone. Big bad El Niño, that horrendous and tenacious storm pattern emanating from cyclical forces dominant to the Pacific Ocean, has gone from splinter to spear, even for the most stoic usually unperturbed by weather. And, as El Niño has wreaked damage from coast to coast, border to border, and actually around the globe, the result has been a substantial loss of the fair weather, including the fair-weather mood, most of us take for granted.

Rarely have so many been so quick to blame every problem — including the chicken virus, Monica-gate, and the fascistic excesses of the IRS — on El Niño. Nevertheless, while accusing a cyclical weather pattern for the end of civilization is clearly a case of overkill, there is something else — for real — that we can lay at the doorstep of this mother-of-all weather dysrhythmias: **Getting fat and being depressed.**

The Origins of SAD
Putting on fat and feeling depressed have a special collusion through two allied syndromes: seasonal affective disorder (SAD) and seasonal affective eating disorder (SAED). SAD and SAED are characterized by recurrent depressions and compulsive eating

behavior that occur annually around the same time period each year. The usual peak for SAD occurs in autumn/winter, usually with full remission following in spring/summer. With approximately the same cycle, SAED involves compulsive eating binges and carbohydrate cravings. Because these disorders overlap — many contend that they are one and the same — we will henceforth refer to them as SAD. SAD is additionally often accompanied by additional symptoms, including:

- fatigue
- sadness
- decreased libido
- hopelessness
- anxiety
- decreased interest in work and social activities
- weight gain
- excessive sleeping
- psychomotor retardation.

Like your typical reaction to the onslaught of bad weather, SAD manifests slowly with garden variety complaints and progresses to full blown mood shifts. The grin-and-bear-it attempt to ignore depressed feelings drifts into hopeless resignation.

The scientific data establishing SAD are significant and unambiguous. Seasonal and environmental influences on depression have been written about for more than 2,000 years.[1] More recently in the mid-1970s researchers examining neuropsychiatric records for England and Wales noted the correspondence between manic depressive persons and the high concentration of births in the early months of the year and a corresponding deficiency in the summer months.[2] When SAD was first described in the early 1980s, it was thought to exist as a subset of bipolar (manic-depressive) disorder and to involve, in addition to over eating and depression, the need for excessive sleep.[3] In the UK, a 72% increase in sleep from around seven hours in the summer to nine in winter was reported for SAD sufferers.[4]

In the later 1980s researchers studying bipolar type II affective disorder subgrouping noticed that this condition included features such as overeating, oversleeping, atypical depression, and seasonal affective disorder. When considered together with an association to several abnormal motivated behaviors such as alcoholism and eating disorders the idea dawned on scientists that a distinct morbid mechanism involving serotonin may underlie it.[5] Serotonin is the major inhibitory neurotransmitter in the brain. Others concluded that there were nutrient imbalances in depressive disorders involving possible brain mechanisms.[6]

Dull Weather Triggers Depression

A weather catastrophe such as the El Niño of 1997-1998, in effect, prolongs the seasons thus making the Winter's SAD activity spill over into Spring. One scientific study's findings suggest that changes in atmospheric temperature played an important role the triggering of Spring-type SAD. Another study found that the depressive episodes of some people may be triggered at any time of the year if the weather is unusually dull, characterized by an unusually low light intensity.[7] Other studies indicate that temperature change alone may bring about SAD.[8] Other studies are in agreement that weather circumstances needed to induce SAD-type reactions include reduced sunshine, global radiation, length of daylight and temperature changes.[9] Such conditions are typical of those fostered by El Niño. However, there is some controversy when analyzing winter depression with regard to cloud cover, rainfall or atmospheric pressure. But the data is clear that for some individuals subject to SAD there is a another trough of symptoms in March/April often equal in severity to that of November/December, and that in particularly inclement weather the trough can get deeper and longer. In some instances, SAD depression can extend — if weather conditions are severe and prolonged enough as is the case with this year's El Niño — right through the entire Spring!

In colder climates Winter SAD is a common condition that increases in prevalence and proportion to the number and darkness of overcast days.[10] A random sample of nearly 300 Alaskans found that over 9.2% met diagnostic criteria for seasonal affective disorder, one of the highest figures yet reported.

These cyclic winter affective disorders occurred more often in women than men (ratio=3:2) and were more prevalent among residents who were younger than 40 years of age.[11]

Light Therapy

One of the more reported clinical practices for SAD has been the use of light therapy, use of which seeks to correct the disturbance of circadian rhythm caused by desynchronization between the solar clock and the human biologic clock during seasons of short photoperiods. These include winter or extended periods of overcast, cloudy, or gloomy weather. Light therapy, also known as phototherapy, is thought to alter the production patterns of melatonin, the neurotransmitter serotonin, and the peptide neurohormone corticotropin releasing hormone (CRH) which together play a pathophysiological role when altered by Winter seasonal affective disorder.[12] For some people phototherapy can help shorten SAD. However, the timing schedule of phototherapy remains controversial, the results are spotty, and therapy is both inconvenient and time consuming. Studies show that going outdoors can be more therapeutic than daylight-emulating artificial light.

St John's Wort

Also believed to be effective with SAD is **St John's wort** (hypericum extract). In one single-blind study 900 mg of St John's wort was given over the course of 4 weeks to two small groups suffering from SAD along with either bright light phototherapy or dim light therapy (placebo) for two hours each day. At the end of the study both groups were found to measure a significant reduction in the total score of the Hamilton Depression Rating Scale.[13] There was no significant difference when bright light therapy was combined with St John's wort, compared to the situation without bright light therapy. St John's wort was well tolerated suggesting that St John's wort may be useful for SAD.[14]

Melatonin Not Effective

Despite the theory behind phototherapy and data showing melatonin to be effective in the treatment of circadian-rhythm related sleep disturbances, studies have demonstrated that melatonin has little to no impact on the depressive symptoms of SAD.[15] Light remains the therapy of choice despite its shortcomings. But recently scientists have identified the common feature of what they believe to be the root of the SAD problem: serotonin depletion,[16] which is related to serotonin deficiency syndrome, a problem about which readers of this publication have heard much.

By the 1980s, scientists had firmed up their understanding of the causal connections between seasonal conditions, the cycles of mood and psychological health. In 1989, a study found that a serotonin-enhancing drug (D-fenfluramine, later of fen-phen infamy) was effective for the affective and appetitive symptoms of SAD.[17] It was possible to say that carbohydrate craving was a kind of substance abuse because certain foods in that category could be eaten specifically for their serotonin-mediated psychotropic effects. This conclusion supported the idea that nutritional deficiencies could upturn the psychological cart and that there was a strong element of neuropsychopharmacological malfunctioning behind seasonal mood swings.

Serotonin and SAD

Central serotonin pathways have been found to play an important role in the modulation of mood and behavioral impulsivity, and regulation of eating patterns, qualitatively and quantitatively. The many studies showing that the amino acids L-tryptophan and 5-hydroxytryptophan, and serotonin potentiating drugs relieve depression disorders suggest that brain serotonin influences pathophysiology. The tryptophans are precursors to the endogenous (inside the body) production of serotonin, the major inhibitory neurotransmitter in the brain. When tryptophan is taken along with carbohydrates the result is an increase in the plasma ratio of tryptophan to other large neutral amino acids, greater concomitant entry into the brain and increased serotonin synthesis. When those with SAD consume excessive carbohydrate intake their actions reflect a self-medication that temporarily relieves the vegetative symptoms via an increased central serotonergic activity.[18]

Using a tryptophan depletion test, it is possible to induce a rapid and substantial lowering of both total and free plasma tryptophan with consequent decreases in brain serotonin content and also cerebral serotonin function. When scientists used this test to measure health subjects with a genetic risk for affective disorder, their condition was worsened by induced tryptophan depletion.[16] This indicates the relevance of altered brain serotonin function in the pathophysiology of affective disorders and strengthens the importance of serotonin to help prevent depressive states.

Tryptophan and 5-Hydroxytryptophan

Because the production and utilization of serotonin appears to be central to alleviating the symptoms of SAD, and because carbohydrate craving is also symptomatic to this syndrome, it appears as if SAD may be viewed as a dietary deficiency with special seasonal considerations given to the Winter months or to other periods of sunshine deprivation. Other special winter dietary considerations have been identified throughout history, not the least of which is vitamin C deficiency (scurvy) which has traditionally been more of a problem in winter, when ascorbate concentrations decline in food and the availability of citrus fruit becomes scarce. Energy requirements also vary according to season and activity levels and we also know that stressor conditions can increase the utilization of noradrenaline and dopamine and thus upset the balance with other neurotransmitters such as serotonin.[21]

Based on the serotonin connection to SAD it stands to reason that 5-hydroxytryptophan (5-HTP) — related to tryptophan and much closer to serotonin (5-HTP is the immediate precursor to serotonin) on the metabolic pathway — would be useful because it is a superior serotonin producer. Indeed, in one study, after 5-HTP was administered orally at 200 mg/d to 26 depressed patients, serum cortisol levels were significantly higher compared with controls.[22] Serum cortisol increase has been found to correlate positively with tests to measure affective disorder and to indicate improvement.

A double-blind study examined the effect of 200 mg oral doses of 5-HTP in ten depressed patients with SAD and ten controls. Before administration of 5-HTP, data disclosed those with SAD had significantly higher basal levels of serum prolactin and a trend toward higher basal levels of serum compared with controls. After administration of 5-HTP, the cortisol level significantly increased and the prolactin level significantly decreased.[23] High levels of prolactin have been shown to reflect many depressive states.

The scientific literature on 5-HTP appears to make it an extremely valuable dietary aid to insure support for a wide spectrum of functional benefits. There is a large variety of literature on the use of this serotonin precursor for conditions associated with serotonin deficiency.[24-49]

Fat Loss Too

Scientific observation has also shown 5-HTP to be associated with diminished appetite, decreased food intake, and weight loss in obese subjects. In one double-blind study, 20 obese people were given either 5-HTP (900 mg/d) or a placebo for two consecutive 6-week periods. Significant weight loss resulted along with reduced carbohydrate intake with continuous levels of satisfaction (satiety) reported.[51]

When 5-HTP was administered to 26 healthy, non-depressed subjects marked mood elevation was observed and the subjects reported feeling happier.[52-53] The authors remarked at how the improved mood changes seemed to increase rather than plateau over the course time during which 5-HTP effects were measured.

Another study followed 247 subjects who fasted on a very-low calorie diet for a 2-year period using a considerably smaller amount of 5-HTP (15 mg/d) along with other nutrients thought to be of value as part of a weight control program.[54] Those chosen for the study were particularly unable to either achieve their desired target weight or maintain it.

The results included considerable decreases in food craving (70% for males and 63% for females) as well as a significant decreases in binge eating (66% for females and 41% for males). Those taking the 5-HTP formulation saw the amount of excessess fat delined by half for men and women alike. At the follow up after the fast, those taking the 5-HTP-containing formulation were found to regain only about 15% of the weight lost vs about 42%

for the control group.

Recently famed thermogenic researcher Astrup has also found that a particular regimen helps prevent regaining weight lost through dieting . The report followed 41 women and 2 men who were obese (with a body mass idex of 27-40) but otherwise healthy on two different weight regimes, one of which was very low calorie and the other a conventional diet.[55] To induce fat burning both groups were given 20 mg of ephedrine and 200 mg caffeine three times daily and followed for one year. The low-calorie group achieved its weight loss goal of about 30 lbs, on average, in eight weeks while the conventional diet group took 17 weeks to lose on average 30 lbs.

Following the weight loss, the subjects entered a 6 to 12 months period of weight maintenance at which the very low calorie group was found to have regained less than 2 lbs for a loss maintenance of nearly 98%. The conventional diet group — surprise! — regained, on average, about 9 lbs for a loss maintenance of 70%. Then another 6 month period followed and the subjects were again measured. The conventional/slow loss group was found to have regained 25 lbs while the very low calorie/fast loss group regained only 12 lbs. Also at follow up, 65% of the very low calorie/fast loss group vs 40% of the conventional/slow loss group has maintained a weight loss greater than 12 lbs.

These data suggest that the rate of initial weight loss has no effect on weight maintenance contrary to the "famine mechanism" that cautions about rapid weight loss for purposes of health. Tripping the cellular setting for famine-level (slower) metabolism explains the yo-yo syndrome in dieting where weight loss is gained back faster and then some. However, this study may indicate that ephedrine and caffeine may allow a person to lose weight faster without setting off metabolic alarms. The subjects in the fast weight loss group lost a little more than 3 lbs per week while the slower group lost a little under 2 lbs per week. Nontheless, we still think it is best to work with a physician when attempting to lose more than 10% of your body weight.

5-HTP Helps Blow El Niño Away

Whether El Niño or any bad weather you may encounter gets you down (in spirit) or up (in weight) or both, it's a good time to decide to do something about it and formulations containing 5-HTP can help. A starting point would be a formulation containing 50 mg of 5-HTP per serving combined with a synergistic amount of St John's wort, magnesium and vitamin B_6. Another way to address El Niño would be a formulation containing 25 mg of 5-HTP per serving along with about 333 mg of ma huang (containing 20 mg of active ephedrine), 65 mg of caffeine, 50 mg of white willow bark, vitamins C and B_6 and chromium aspartate. Formulations such as these might be used together, the first containing 5-HTP and St. John's wort at bedtime and the second with 5-HTP and ephedra about an hour before meals. For some individuals, formulations containing ephedrine may not be suitable. Please consult with your doctor before initiating any program containing 5-HTP and St. John's wort or ephedra.

Whatever your choice, whether you're SAD, pre-SAD, or post-SAD, it's possible to get out of the cycles of mood shift and uncontrolled cravings and 5-HTP products can help. Wouldn't you rather be happy than SAD?

References

1. Wehr TA, Rosenthal NE. Seasonality and affective illness. *Am J Psychiatry.* 1989;146:829-839.
2. Hare EH. Manic-depressive psychosis and season of birth. *Acta Psychiatr. Scand.* 1975;52:69-79.
3. Rosenthal NE, Sack DA, Gillin JC, Lewy AJ, Goodwin FK, Davenport Y, Mueller PS, Newsome DA, Wehr TA. Seasonal affective disorder. A description of the syndrome and preliminary findings with light therapy. *Arch Gen Psychiatry.* 1984;41:72-80.
4. Ford K. A seasonal depression. Management of seasonal affective disorder. *Prof Nurse.* 1992;8:94-98.
5. DePaulo Jr JR, Simpson SG. Therapeutic and genetic prospects of an atypical affective disorder. *J Clin Psychopharmacol.* 1987;7(6 Suppl):50S-54S.
6. Wurtman RJ, O'Rourke D, Wurtman JJ. Nutrient imbalances in depressive disorders. Possible brain mechanisms. *Ann N Y Acad Sci.* 1989;575:75-82.
7. Summers L, Shur E. The relationship between onsets of depression and sudden drops in solar irradiation. *Biol Psychiatry.* 1992;32:1164-1172.
8. Wehr TA, Sack DA, Rosenthal NE. Seasonal affective disorder with summer

depression and winter hypomania. *Am J Psychiatry.* 1987;144:1602-1603.

9. Molin J, Mellerup E, Bolwig T, Scheike T, Dam H. The influence of climate on development of winter depression. *J Affect Disord.* 1996;37:151-155.

10. Dilsaver SC, Jaeckle RS. The naturally occurring rhythm of blues: winter depression. *Ohio Med.* 1990;86:58-61.

11. Booker JM, Hellekson CJ. Prevalence of seasonal affective disorder in Alaska. *Am J Psychiatry.* 1992;149:1176-1182.

12. Wehr TA. Seasonal vulnerability to depression. Implications for etiology and treatment. *Encephale.* 1992;18 (Spec No 4):479-483.

13. Martinez B, Kasper S, Ruhrmann S, Moller HJ. Hypericum in the treatment of seasonal affective disorders. *J Geriatr Psychiatry Neurol.* 1994;7(Suppl 1):S29-S33.

14. Kasper S. Treatment of seasonal affective disorder (SAD) with hypericum extract. *Pharmacopsychiatry.* 1997;30(Suppl 2):89-93.

15. Wirz-Justice A, Graw P, Krauchi K, Gisin B, Arendt J, Aldhous M, Poldinger W. Morning or night-time melatonin is ineffective in seasonal affective disorder. *J Psychiatr Res.* 1990;24(2):129-137.

16. Neumeister A, Praschak-Rieder N, Hesselmann B, Tauscher J, Kasper S. The tryptophan depletion test. Basic principles and clinical relevance. *Nervenarzt.* 1997;68:556-56.

17. Wurtman RJ, O'Rourke D, Wurtmann JJ. Nutrient imbalances in depressive disorders. Possible brain mechanisms. *Ann N Y Acad Sci.* 1989;575:75-82.

18. Moller SE. Serotonin, carbohydrates, and atypical depression. *Pharmacol. Toxicol.* 1992;71(Suppl 1):61-71.

19. McGrath RE, Buckwald B, Resnick EV. The effect of L-tryptophan on seasonal affective disorder. *J Clin Psychiatry.* 1990;51:162-163.

20. Lam RW, Levitan RD, Tam EM, Yatham LN, Lamoureux S, Zis AP. L-tryptophan augmentation of light therapy in patients with seasonal affective disorder. *Can J Psychiatry.* 1997;42:303-306.

21. Roth KA, Mefford IM, Barchas JD. Epinephrine, norepinephrine, dopamine and serotonin: differential effects of acute and chronic stress on regional brain amines. *Brain Res.* 1982;239:417-424.

22. Meltzer HY, Perline R, Tricou BJ, Lowy M, Robertson A. Effect of 5-hydroxytryptophan on serum cortisol levels in major affective disorders. II. Relation to suicide, psychosis, and depressive symptoms. *Arch Gen Psychiatry.* 1984;41:379-387.

23. Jacobsen FM, Sack DA, Wehr TA, Rogers S, Rosenthal NE. Neuroendocrine response to 5-hydroxytryptophan in seasonal affective disorder. *Arch Gen Psychiatry.* 1987;44:1086-1091.

24. Laboucarie J, Rascol A, Guiraud-Chaumeil B, El-Hage W. La place du 5-hydroxytryptophane levogyre dans les etats depressifs. *Rev Med.* 1977;13:519-524.

25. Takahashi S, Kondo H, Kato N. Effect of L-5-hydroxytryptophan on brain monoamine metabolism and evaluation of its clinical effect in depressed patients. *J Psychiat Res.* 1975;12:177-187.

26. van Praag H, Lemus C. Monamine precursors in the treatment of psychiatric disorders. In: Wurtman R, Wurtman J, eds. *Food Constitutents Affecting Normal and Abnormal Behavior: Nutrition and the Brain.* New

York: Raven Press; 1986:80-138.

27. van Praag H, Van Den Burg W, Bos E, Dols L. 5-hydroxytryptophan in combination with clomipramine in "therapy-resistant" depression. *Psychopharmacology.* 1974;38:267-269.

28. Nardini M, DeStefano R, Ianuccelli M, Borghesi R, Battistini N. Treatment of depression with L-5-hydroxytryptophan combined with chlorimipramine: A double-blind study. *J Clin Pharmacol Res.* 1983;3:239-250.

29. Angst J, Woggon B, Schoopf J. The treatment of depression with L-5-hydroxytryptophan versus imipramine: Results of two open and one double-blind study. *Arch Psychiatr Nervenkr.* 1977;224:175-186.

30. Pöldinger W, Calanchini B, Schwarz W. A functional-dimensional approach to depression: serotonin deficiency as a target syndrome in a comparison of 5-hydroxytryptophan and fluvoxamine. *Psychopathology.* 1991;24:53-81.

31. Kahn R, Westenberg H. L-5-Hydroxytryptophan in the treatment of anxiety disorders. *J Affect Disord.* 1985;8:197-200.

32. Den Boer J, Westenberg H. Behavioral, neuroendocrine, and biochemical effects of 5-hydroxytryptophan administration in panic disorder. *Psychiatry Res.* 1990;31:267-278.

34. Soulairac A, Lambinet H. Action du 5-hydroxytryptophane, precurseur de la serotonine sur les troubles du sommeil. *Ann Med-Psychol.* 1977;135:792-798.

35. Ursin R. The effect of 5-hydroxytryptophan and L-tryptophan on wakefulness and sleep patterns in the cat. *Brain Res.* 1976;106:106-115.

37. Blundell J. Pharmacological approaches to appetite suppression. *Trends Pharmacol.* 1991;12:147-157.

38. Cangiano C, Ceci F, Cascino A, et al. Eating behavior and adherence to dietary prescriptions in obese subjects treated with 5-hydroxytryptophan. *Am J Clin Nutr.* 1992;56:863-868.

39. Titus F, Davalos A, Alom J, Codina A. 5-Hydroxytryptophan versus methysergide in the prophylaxis of migraine. Randomized clinical trial. *Eur Neurol.* 1986;25:327-329.

40. De Benedittis G, Massei R. 5-HTP precursors in migraine prophylaxis: A double-blind crossover study with L-5-hydroxytryptophan versus placebo. *Clin J Pain.* 1986;3:123-129.

41. Pratt L, Ford D, Crum R, Armenian H, Gallo J, Eaton W. Depression, psychotropic medication, and risk of myocardial infarction: Prospective data from the Baltimore ECA follow-up. *Circulation.* 1996;94:3123-3129.

42. Avery D, Winokur G. Mortality in depressed patients treated with electroconvulsive therapy and antidepressants. *Arch Gen Psychiatry.* 1976;33:1029-1037.

43. Carney R, Rich M, Tevelde A, Saini J, Clark K, Jaffe A. Major depressive disorder in coronary artery disease. *Am J Cardiol.* 1987;60:1273-1275.

44. Hance C, Carney R, Freedland K, Skala J. Depression in patients with coronary heart disease: A 12-month follow-up. *Gen Hosp Psychiatry.* 1996;18:61-65.

45. Carney R, Rich M, Freedland K, et al. Major depressive disorder predicts cardiac events in patients with coronary artery disease. *Psychosom. Med.*

1988;50:723-627.
46. Barefoot J, Schroll M. Symptoms of depression, acute myocardial infarction, and total mortality in a community sample. *Circulation.* 1996;93:1976-1980.
47. Carney R, Saunders R, Freedland K, Stein P, Rich M, Jaffe A. Association of depression with reduced heart rate variability in coronary artery disease. *Am J Cardiol.* 1995;76:562-564.
48. Jonas S, Franks P, Ingram D. Are symptoms of anxiety and depression risk factors for hypertension? *Arch Fam Med.* 1997;6:43-49.
49. Frimerman A, Miller H, Lanaido S, Keren G. Changes in hemostatic function at times of cyclic variation in occupational stress. *Am J Cardiol.* 1997;79:72-75.
50. Puhringer W, Wiz-Justice A, Graw P, Lacoste V, Gastpar M. Intravenous L-5-hydroxytryptophan in normal subjects: an interdisciplinary precursor loading study. Part 1: Implications of reproducible mood elevation. *Pharmakopsychiatr Neuropsychopharmakol.* 1976;9:260-268.
51. Cangiano C, Ceci F, Cascino A, Del Ben M, Laviano A, Muscaritoli M, Antonucci F, Rossi-Fanelli F. Eating behavior and adherence to dietary prescriptions in obese adult subjects treated with 5-hydroxytryptophan. *Am J Clin Nutr.* 1992;56:863-867.
52. Trimble M, Chadwick D, Reynolds EH, Marsden CD. Letter: L 5-Hydroxytryptophan and mood. *Lancet.* 1975;1(7906):583.
53. Trimble M, Chadwick D, Reynolds EH, Marsden CD. Letter: L 5-Hydroxytryptophan and mood. *Lancet.* 1975;1(7906):583.
54. Blum K, Cull JG, Chen TJH, Garcia-Swan S, Holder J,M, Wood R, Braverman ER,. Bucci LR, Trachtenberg M.C Clinical evidence for effectiveness of PhenCal(TM) in maintaining weight loss in an open-label, controlled, 2-year study. *Current Therapeutic Research - Clinical and Experimental.* 1997;58:745-763.
55. Toubro S; Astrup A. Randomized comparison of diets for maintaining obese subjects' weight after major weight loss: ad lib, low fat, high carbohydrate diet v fixed energy intake. *BMJ.* 1997;314:29-34.

CHAPTER 17

Q&A

Who's Who
WB = Will Block
GV = Dr. Gail Valentine

Natural 5-HTP: Know the Difference

Q: I was going to order 5-HTP from you, but I got concerned about its safety, when I read an article claiming it is risky. Why are there so many discrepancies between what you say and what they say? I have enclosed the article for you so you can respond. Please let me know because I am still interested in this product.

AB

A: Bear in mind that the article you sent limits assessment, since there are no references listed. However, it seems to be saying, firstly, that if pure 5-HTP were available for sale, then it might be worthwhile to use it in the same manner that tryptophan was once used. Secondly, a highly selective enzymatic process is required to produce pure 5-HTP. The article implies that a non-enzymatic process, meaning certain synthetic processes, may produce by-products that are slightly different versions of 5-HTP and these slightly different versions could possibly be neurotoxic to serotonin neurons and receptors.

This means that the enzymatic process produces 5-HTP and only 5-HTP while the synthetic process may produce slightly different versions of 5-HTP, which can be toxic. In addition, the article says that this enzymatic process occurs in the body, which the reader could interpret in context as only in the body. Actually the enzymatic process of producing 5-HTP and nothing but 5-HTP also occurs as a natural biological process within the plant, *griffonia simplicifolia*. Some of the best manufacturers purchase 5-HTP derived only from the *griffonia* plant, which is therefore free from possible neurotoxins (unlike some synthetic processes) and therefore pure, safe, and worthwhile taking for similar purposes as tryptophan.

The article also went on to talk about the tryptophan contamination of 1989, which caused a number of deaths (when a Japanese company changed important manufacturing procedures). The article seems to be implying to watch out for synthetic 5-HTP, because it could end up doing the same thing as the tryptophan contamination. Consequently, if a manufacturer is sure to buy only the highest quality of raw materials and uses only plant-derived 5-HTP, the above comment is superfluous.

Lastly, the article also states that "commercially available 5-HTP is not produced enzymatically." This statement implies that all 5-HTP available for purchase by any manufacturer is a non-enzymatic 5-HTP product, meaning it is a synthetic. But much of the 5-HTP available for consumption comes directly from a natural source, the plant *griffonia simplicifolia*. Therefore, it is enzymatically produced (in the plant), and its commercially available appears to make the above statement altogether false.

Why so many discrepancies? One possible explanation is that in the editing process of a publication/article, certain statements standing alone may be factual, but not necessarily complete or true in the whole picture.

Dr GV

No More Restless Nights
Testimonial: I am very glad to know that I can continue to take 5-HTP. I find it much easier to take 5-HTP once a day instead of St. John's wort and inositol twice a day. I even got my husband to start 5-HTP about a month ago. He had very restless nights and couldn't wake up in the morning. Now his sleep is much more rested. He has even mentioned 5-HTP to co-workers who he feels are under a lot of stress and may be having sleepless nights. Thanks for a very safe and natural product.

JF

5-HTP Only at Bedtime?
Q: Do you recommend taking 5-HTP only at bedtime? Are there other times during the day which are advisable?

CJ

A Suggested use as indicated on the bottle is that you may take 1 to 4 servings at bedtime which is equivalent to 50 mg to 200 mg. I find that most people seem to do well on simply 25 mg to 100 mg at bedtime, although there are others who take daytime amounts of 25 mg to 100 mg up to three times per day (including the bedtime amount) with good results.

Remember that 5-HTP can make you feel relaxed or drowsy. Therefore you should be cautious about your activities. Do not drive or operate machinery or the like until you know how your own body is going to respond. I recommend starting with small amounts (12.5 mg to 25 mg) during the daytime and increasing as, and if, needed.

Dr GV

5-HTP and the Fen-Phen Tragedy

Q: I have been taking a 5-HTP formulation for 7 months. I have had great success. However, I read something alarming in my local newspaper. The article was about fen/phen causing heart valve disease due to increased levels of serotonin. I certainly do not want to help one problem only to create another.

GP

A: It is true that there have been recent discoveries in long-term users of the weight loss products, fen-phen (fenfluramine and phentermine) and Redux® (dexfenfluramine), with regard to valvular heart disease. Some of these patients have been found to have elevated levels of serum serotonin. Elevated serotonin is a correlation and is not known to be causal. But a likely explanation of the problem is that the drugs in question prevent expended, damaged, or functionally altered serotonin from being expunged from the body.

Even so, it must be noted that 5-HTP is not serotonin. The brain essentially provides an "escape hatch" where 5-HTP is absorbed from the peripheral bloodstream and crosses the blood-brain barrier. It is in the brain where the bulk of the conversion of 5-HTP to serotonin takes place. And this is a good thing, because this is exactly where the serotonin is needed. 5-HTP is not a "new kid on the block" nor is it a xenobiotic (a substance alien to the body), as is the case with both Redux and fenfluramine. More than 4,000 studies have been published on 5-HTP over the last three decades, and I cannot find a single incidence cited where ingesting 5-HTP has caused any serious side effects, including valvular heart disease.

Dr GV

Is 5-HTP Expensive?

Q: I've been using 5-HTP — I like it very much — but why does it have to be so expensive?

EF

A: 5-hydroxytryptophan is in short supply because it is a natural product, not yet commercial synthesized. So it may seem expensive. However, when compared to related products it really isn't so expensive: A low range dose of 5 HTP (50 mg) is about the same price as a low range dose of tryptophan (500 mg) — ie, when tryptophan was available. Also, 5-HTP activity is synergistic when used with vitamin B$_6$ and St. John's wort. A formulation of these items would be the most economical. Finally, compare the cost of 5 HTP to some pharmaceuticals (like Prozac, Zoloft, Paxil, etc.), and you'll find that it begins to look like a bargain.

WB

Growth Hormone Release

Q: Does 5-HTP release growth hormone like tryptophan does?

KP

A: A significant effect on growth hormone release in humans after oral ingestion of 2 grams of L tryptophan has been demonstrated.[1] I would expect a similar rise with 50-100 mg of 5-HTP. Furthermore, there is evidence that melatonin may enhance growth hormone secretion,[2-3] and 5 HTP is a precursor of serotonin and melatonin. So although the data are not conclusive with regard to tryptophan and growth hormone, I believe that tryptophan and 5-HTP probably significantly enhance the release of growth hormone in humans.

Dr GV

References
1. Hyyppa MT, Jolma T, Liira J, Langvik VA, Kytomaki O. L-tryptophan treatment and the episodic secretion of pituitary hormones and cortisol. *Psychoneuroendocrinology* 1979;4:29-35.
2. Smythe, G.A., and Lazarus, L. Growth hormone regulation by melatonin

. . . .
and serotonin. *Nature* 1973;244:230-231.
3. Valcavi R, Zini M, Maestroni G, and Conti A. Melatonin stimulates growth hormone secretion through pathways other than the growth-hormone releasing hormone. *Clinical Endocrinology* 1993;39:193-199.

Calming Kids With 5-HTP?

Q: Is 5-HTP OK to give to kids as a calming agent?

PS

A: We do not generally endorse the use of supplements for children, in part because there are usually few studies that use children as "experimental" subjects (remember Nuremberg and the idea that non-consenters should not be used for medical experiments?*) and primarily because of the litigious age in which we live. We believe that it is best to consult with your family health-care professional before introducing any such items to your children's regimen.

Be that as it may, we offer the following information to be drawn to the attention of your health care professional. SSRIs have been reported in the literature to be of benefit for conditions of depression and obsessive-compulsive disorder with generally good results.[1] 5-HTP has reported to be beneficial for adults, and compared favorably to an SSRI in treating these same conditions.

An Italian study involving 48 elementary and junior high school students found 5-HTP to be beneficial for recurring headache and sleep disorders.[2] Of particular interest was the effect of 5 HTP on memory deficiencies for otherwise normally intelligent students. Performance was improved.

WB

1. DeVane CL, Sallee FR. Serotonin selective reuptake inhibitors in child and adolescent psychopharmacology: A review of published experience. *J Clin Psyc* 1996;57:55-66.
2. De Giorgis G, Miletto R. Iannuccelli M. et al. Headache in association with sleep disorder in children: A psychodiagnostic evaluation and controlled clinical study: L 5-HTP versus placebo. *Drugs Exp Clin Res* 1987;13:425-433.

---

* Apparently the FDA does not remember. As per the agency's new rule, patients may be "granted" experimental emergency treatments without their consent whenever an independent physician and the local institutional review board agree that the need of a trial "address a life threatening situation" and "available treatments are unproven or unsatisfactory." Sounds almost good, until you think about it. The FDA has been the greatest obstructionist agency in existence to medical and bio-medical progress. Who would be crazy enough to want to give the FDA the power to violate the individual's autonomy in the name of "we know best?" The quick answer is: those who abjure freedom and dignity.

Will 5-HTP Lower Sex Drive?

Q: Will 5-HTP lower my sex drive because of serotonin's conflict with dopamine?

CM

A: The effects of serotonin on sex drive is directly related to the relative amount (as is the case with most compounds) and especially to the type of serotonergic receptors that are stimulated. In rat studies, stimulation of the 5-HT1 receptors increases sexual facilitation, and stimulation of 5-HT2 receptors produces sexual inhibition.[1] In a particular study with male rats, 5-HTP produced an increased number of mounts and intromissions to ejaculation. When the lab animals were pretreated with benserazide, a carboxylase inhibitor that causes serotonin production to decrease peripherally and to increase in the brain, there was a further delay in the length of time to ejaculation. [This might be positive depending on the state of your libido.] The effect of 25 mg of 5-HTP delivered intraperitoneally to female rats reduced lordosis, or sexual posturing. This is the equivalent of many times this amount given orally for a human.

Rest assured that the amount of 5-HTP needed to reduce the sex drive is large, and that according to one study, the subthreshold was 12.5 mg/kg of body weight for rats. All other things equal, this would translate to about 850 mg of 5-HTP for a 150 lb human.[2] Since "garden variety" deficiency-syndrome usage is 50 to 200 mg, sexual inhibition is unlikely to occur.

WB

References
1. Ahlenius S, Larsson K. Opposite effects of 5-methoxy-N,N-di-methyl-tryptamine and 5 hydroxytryptophan on male rat sexual behavior. *Pharmacol Biochem Behav* 1991;38:201-205.
2. Fernandez-Guasti A, Rodriguez-Manzo G. Further evidence showing that the inhibitory action of serotonin on rat masculine Sexual behavior is mediated after the stimulation of 5-HT1B receptors. *Pharmacol Biochem Behav* 1992; 42:529-533.

5-HTP/St. John's Wort Combo

Q: Why would a person take St. John's wort along with 5-HTP, and why so much less St. John's wort than in a usual serving size?

YT

A: For two reasons: St. John's wort is a mild "garden variety" antidepressant, and also a mild MAO inhibitor (MAOI). Its antidepressant characteristics are thought to be independent of its MAO inhibition. In the past (and still to a minor degree) MAOIs have been used for depression, but their use has fallen out of favor with the rise of tricyclics, and more recently SSRIs (like Prozac). However, MAOIs work by reducing the ability of monoamine oxidase to clear neurotransmitters from the brain. Thus, neurotransmitters such as serotonin will operate with an added degree of endurance or attenuation.

Thirty mcg of St. John's wort's active ingredient, hypericin, used with 50 mg of 5-HTP has been found to produce an enhancement plateau at which buffering is optimized. Using too much St. John's wort along with 5 HTP can frequently have a stimulatory effect which may not be desirable, especially given the goals of use. St. John's wort (or products containing it) should not be used by anyone taking MAOIs.

Otherwise, within the ranges of the amounts used in the research, there are few side effects from St. John's wort. Negative affects may arise from the high doses that have been used for its antiviral activity in the treatment of AIDS-related conditions.

WB

St. John's Wort OK with 5-HTP?
Q: I am taking St John's wort (900 mg daily) for depression. Is it advisable to also take 5-HTP?

CP

A: I am assuming that you are taking 300 mg of a 0.3 percent extract three times per day which means you should be getting 2.7 mg of hypericin per day. Since you are already at the high end of the amount recommended for hypericin and still are considering adding 5-HTP, I am wondering if you are getting results.

I can find no studies where hypericin and 5-HTP were administered concomitantly. There are anecdotal reports of hyperactive or "racey" feelings for some people when taking hypericin and 5-HTP together at their usual/recommended amounts. Reducing the amount of one or the other or both substances seems a rational approach.

Formulations which contain a standard amount of 5-HTP (50 mg/tsp or cap) with a very small amount of hypericin (30mcg/tsp or cap) have been reported to be more appropriate. The significantly smaller amount of hypericin tends to eliminate the undesirable effects of combination use while enhancing the positive impact of the 5-HTP. Straight 5-HTP capsules without any hypericin will also work but not as well for some people.

There are multiple studies that have shown 5-HTP to be beneficial for a wider range of uses. When compared to the more limited outcomes in studies using St John's wort, 5-HTP is by far, more beneficial for serotonin deficiency syndrome. It is difficult to advise what would be just the right approach for you, not knowing your age or your medical history, among many other factors. I would recommend that if you are considering combining different therapies you should be supervised by your physician. For more information on St John's wort seek out Dr. Ray Sahelian's book on the subject.

Dr GV

How Much St. John's Wort?
Q: How much St. John's wort can a person take with 5-HTP?

IP

A: It is inadvisable to take large amounts of St. John's wort with any neurotransmitter precursor formulation because of the possibility of excessive stimulation. This is also true of any one of number of combinations such as phenylalanine and coffee. By all means, if a 5-HTP/St. John's wort formulation by itself produces restlessness or insomnia, cut down on the amount, at first by halving the serving size. If restlessness continues, do not continue to use 5-HTP or St. John's wort. You may be sensitive to St. John's wort or 5-HTP itself, or may respond in a paradoxical (opposite to the expected) fashion! It has long been noted that tryptophan, the earlier biochemical pathway precursor to serotonin, causes the opposite effect in some individuals, and the same thing may occur in some people with 5-HTP, however rare.

WB

5-HTP With Other Nutrients

Q: Can you mix 5-HTP with arginine, acetyl L-carnitine (ALC) or "smart drink" formulations?

FL

A: Yes, with certain qualifications. If you are taking 5-HTP at bedtime, you may not want the added energy that ALC or a smart drink provides, since it might interfere with sleep. You must decide for yourself what works best for you. Please let us know your experiences.

WB

5-HTP With Other Antidepressants

Q: Can 5-HTP be used with SSRIs such as Prozac or other antidepressants?

EK

A: One should be cautious about using 5-HTP together with these drugs. There is a condition known as serotonin syndrome which has been found to be caused by mixing serotonin-enhancing drugs together, and there is some suggestion that this might be true for combining tryptophan or 5-HTP with such drugs. If you are using these medications, and wish to add 5-HTP or tryptophan, you should first consult with your healthcare professional.

WB

I believe that 5-HTP-containing products can be used safely with SSRIs (like Prozac, Paxil, etc). I believe that 5-HTP-containing products act more physiologically; thus they are inherently safer than SSRIs. 5-HTP will enhance the effects of SSRIs, and may allow the SSRI dose to be reduced or discontinued. However, it is necessary that anyone contemplating changing their medication dosage do so in cooperation with their physician.

With regard to whether formulations containing 5-HTP can be taken with MAOIs, I believe that this caution is also not an absolute contraindication. For example, many people who take 5-HTP are also taking Deprenyl (a MAO-B inhibitor) without ill-effects. And St. John's wort, as stated in the answer above, is also a MAOI. Certainly most people have had no untoward effects with this apparent synergistic combination of supplements.

Dr GV

How Much 5-HTP Should I Take?

Q: All of the studies that you cite use several hundred milligrams of 5-HTP. Why do your products contain only 50 mg/serving?

GK

A: While we point to the literature with all the indicated wider possibilities, our principle thrust in advocating the use of 5-HTP is for "serotonin deficiency syndrome" and for improved mental and memory functioning. Addressing your functional/structural needs may also yield other benefits, but we leave those concerns to you and your healthcare professional. Moreover, a growing body of anecdotal evidence indicates that 50 mg is an adequate level of supplementation for most "garden variety" users. Less is not necessarily better . . . but it's the best starting point to determine your ideal levels. If you know that you're particularly sensitive to supplements, use a powdered form of 5-HTP, preferably as a formulation containing vitamin B_6 and St. John's wort, and start at an even lower level, say 25 mg.

The powder drink mix form will also enable you to take amounts larger than 50 mg, so you do not have to be limited strictly to 50 mg.

WB

Switching Over

Q: I'm taking tryptophan now, but would like to switch over to 5-HTP. How much should I take?

HI

A: Many people find that 50-100 mg of 5-HTP is the equivalent of about 500-1,000 mg of tryptophan. If using a 5-HTP formulation, with cofactors such as vitamin B_6 and St. John's wort, a serving containing only 50 mg or less of 5-HTP may be sufficient.

WB

Low-Level Servings

Q: Why do some 5-HTP studies show dose levels of 500 mg, and most companies only sell it in the amount of 50 mg?

TT

A: We recommend 5-HTP for supplemental "garden variety" use, not as a cure or treatment for disease; thus, the lower amounts of 5-HTP per serving. See the above answer for correspondent levels to tryptophan or straight 5-HTP use.

WB

Amounts Used in Study

Q: How much of each substance was taken in the Pöldinger study?

SB

A: The Pöldinger study cited in *Life Enhancement's* November 1996 issue [and reprinted within this publication] compared the effect of an SSRI against 5-HTP.[1] The amount of 5-HTP was 100 mg, 3 times per day, and the amount of the SSRI fluvoxamine was 50 mg, 3 times/day. [See chart on page 39 for other study amounts.]

WB

References

1. Pöldinger W, Calanchini B, Schwarz W. A functional-dimensional approach to depression: serotonin deficiency as a target syndrome in a comparison of 5-hydroxytryptophan and fluvoxamine. *Psychopathology.* 1991;24:53-81.

5-HTP With Meals?

Q: May 5-HTP be taken with meals?

SD

A: For weight control, it is probably best to take 5-HTP one hour before meals because of the appetite-satisfying characteristics. Taking 5-HTP with food may interfere with optimal bioavailability thus lessening serotonin production because of blood-brain barrier transport competition with other amino acids.

WB

Testimonial: Being involved in the area of holistic healing and alternative medicine, I ran across your supplemental natural hormone therapies. For 3 years I have sold your products to my clients/patients. I wanted to write to you to tell you how great 5-HTP combined with ephedra is. I have 5 clients who swear by its thermogenic effects and its ability to naturally curb ones appetite. I have seen 5-10 pounds of weight loss with clients in a 30-day period without their need for significant dietary change. This has also helped my obese clients to get an edge on their program so that exercise is more comfortable and natural feeling. Keep up the great work! Help us promote happy, healthy, positive, and energetic people!

MR, PhD

5-HTP for Insomnia May Take a Few Weeks
Q: I tried 5-HTP for two nights and did not get relief from my insomnia. What else can you suggest?

MB

A: A little background information first: studies have shown that 5-HTP and SSRI (selective serotonin reuptake inhibitor) drugs such as Prozac to have similar efficacies. One study even tested an SSRI directly against 5-HTP and found the results equivalent — except that 5-HTP had fewer side effects! Both 5-HTP and SSRIs increase the availability of serotonin in the brain yet work in different ways. SSRIs prevent serotonin from being taken up into the neuron, thereby leaving more serotonin available (for reuse). Whereas 5-HTP, as a precursor to serotonin, replenishes brain serotonin.

SSRI drugs, like Prozac, were originally developed to treat depression. Now they are widely prescribed for other disorders, including anxiety, sleep disturbance, chronic migraine headaches, PMS, obesity, and chronic back pain. It is standard to take SSRIs, like Prozac, for at least 4 weeks before determining if they are effective or not. If a person took Prozac for only two days, this would not be an adequate trial of its efficacy.

Similarly, 5-HTP may need more than two days to judge whether it is working. It is not like a prescription sleeping pill that is supposed to knock you out. In the case of sleep disturbance, it is a natural substance to the body for enhancing one's quality of sleep. Most 5-HTP studies have required four to twelve weeks to reach peak benefit levels. In order to give 5-HTP an adequate chance to help you, you may need to take it for a longer time period.

Dr GV

5-HTP for Fibromyalgia

Q: Fibromyalgia has been an ongoing problem for me. I have been coping reasonably well but would mostly like to increase and enhance my quality of sleep. Can I take 5-HTP for this?

BC

A: Fibromyalgia is a commonly encountered disorder characterized by widespread musculoskeletal pain, stiffness, parasthesias (abnormal skin sensations), nonrestorative sleep, and easy fatigability, along with multiple tender points. It occurs mostly in women and usually the women are over 50 years old. It is difficult to diagnose by objective means and diagnosis usually relies on subjective symptoms. Some studies have suggested that the brain neurotransmitter, serotonin, when deficient, may be involved in the pathogenesis of fibromyalgia. Many other studies, by the way, have associated serotonin deficiency with depression, a condition that tends to be more common among those with fibromyalgia than the general population.

Since 5-HTP makes more serotonin available in your brain, this supplement might be something that might be of interest to you based on the fibromyalgia alone.

But in your case it seems you might benefit in more than just one way. In the case of sleep disturbance, which is not an uncommon complaint for fibromyalgia sufferers, 5-HTP has shown to give improvement.

To explain further: tryptophan is the precursor to 5-HTP (5 hydroxytryptophan) and 5-HTP converts to serotonin in the brain. One of the main reasons people used to use tryptophan before its prohibition was to enhance their sleep. One of serotonin's metabolic pathways leads directly to melatonin, widely acknowledged today as the hormone that helps determine our sleep-wake cycle. 5-HTP is one step closer to serotonin. By increasing your serotonin levels by taking 5-HTP you may be increasing your production of melatonin.

5-HTP may be multi-beneficial for you. However, since you have a medical problem, you may want to be advised by your health care provider. There are many things that can cause sleep disturbance and many other things that can mimic the symptoms or complaints of fibromyalgia.

Dr GV

. . . .

5-HTP: Lower-Dosage May Suffice

Q: I have just started taking 5-HTP for its anti-depressant effects. I am starting with a dose of 150 mg in divided doses. My immediate reaction is I feel worse, not better. My concentration is poorer and I feel slightly dazed. I have tried SSRIs in the past and had similar effects for 2 to 3 weeks before they started to work. Should I persevere with 5-HTP?

NM

A My initial reaction to your question is that 150 mg may be too high a beginning dose for you. Many people do well on only 50 mg/day and some do well on even less, 25 mg/day. Also, since 5-HTP can give a relaxed or drowsy affect, it is not surprising that if you are taking it during waking hours that you are experiencing a lack of alertness and clarity. Taking it at bedtime is the standard recommendation, although there are some people who do benefit from it in divided doses throughout the day without without any untoward effects.

As a word of caution, always keep in mind that you may have a medical condition that may require evaluation and monitoring by a physician.

Dr GV

Does St. John's Wort Have a Synergistic Effect?

Q: I have heard that one shouldn't take St. John's wort together with 5-HTP; that the combination is too powerful. Can this be done?

TW

A Yes. I personally find that a 5-HTP formulation containing vitamin B$_6$ and a low level of St. John's wort is much stronger than 5-HTP alone. When I first experimented with 5-HTP alone I needed to take 100-200 mg to feel anything. Yet with the synergistic formulation anything over 50 mg is way too much — I end up still feeling groggy in the morning. This occurs also when I use too much St. John's wort; 30 mg of the 0.3 percent seems about right. I've heard that some people who are very depressed can take higher levels of St John's wort without the racy response that others and myself experience.

However, as with melatonin, the response appears to be highly individual. You must determine the right amount for yourself.

WB

MAO Inhibition From St. John's Wort?

Q: Why combine St. John's wort with 5-HTP? Doesn't its role as an MAO inhibitor preclude usage for some individuals?

DC

A: St. John's wort has antidepressant benefits, apparently independent of its mild MAO aspects, which should not cause a problem any more than the use of deprenyl — an MAO-B, rather than A type inhibitor — should. It is not the fact that it is an MAO inhibitor, but we don't recommend it for people with kidney disease, because of its magnesium content. There are many metabolic abnormalities that can occur in people with kidney problems, particularly with some of the minerals such as potassium, sodium, and magnesium.

WB & Dr GV

Mood Elevation Without Side Effects

Testimonial: I am writing regarding the use of 5-HTP with St. John's wort and vitamin B$_5$. I have been using such a formulation for 2 months now, in place of Paxil,® which I had been prescribed to treat anxiety and minor depression for 2 years. I find that 200 mg daily of 5-HTP is not only a comparable treatment for my symptoms, but it is actually much better. Where Paxil kept my mood from dipping below a certain level, I find under 5-HTP my mood to be elevated beyond what I experienced on 15 mg of Paxil without the sensation of speediness or sexual dysfunction.

A minor concern about your 5-HTP regards your advertisement for it. "The Biochemical Equivalent of a Trip to Hawaii" might suggest to some groups that 5-HTP creates an experience more akin to illicit drugs. I would hate for some groups, government or social, to misconstrue the effects and benefits of this substance and lobby for its scheduling by the government, thereby making it unavailable for those of us who do know how to use it. Words and phrases like "neurotransmitters" and "states of mind" are red flags. We have seen what negative press and sensationalist claims have done to GHB.

I continue to monitor and research the use of nootropics and am excited by their promise. I look forward to the next issue of your magazine to see what new progress has been made with these wonderful articles.

RW

Can Prozac be Used with 5-HTP?

Q: I am taking Prozac. I have been advised by my physician that I should not take any substances in the monoamine oxidase inhibition (MAOI) class. I understand that when St. John's wort is used in conjunction with 5-HTP there may be a weak MAO inhibitor effect. Is there any problem taking Prozac at the same time?

TE

A: Prozac is in a class of antidepressants known as SSRIs (selective serotonin reuptake inhibitors) that have a different mechanism of action than MAO inhibitors. Your physician is correct in advising you not to take MAO inhibitors at the same time.

Although St. John's wort does, in fact, have a weak MAOI effect, I am aware of many people taking both SSRIs, St. John's wort, and 5-HTP without any problems. Of greater concern is the possibility of excessive levels of serotonin in the brain when 5-HTP is combined with an SSRI like Prozac. I have found that most people can reduce or eliminate their SSRIs by judicious titration of 5-HTP, St. John's wort or both. Because the dosage adjustment is somewhat tricky, however, I recommend that patients on Prozac or other SSRIs alter their dosages only under the supervision of their physicians.

Dr GV

5-HTP, MAO Inhibitors and Choline

Q: What about the use of pain killers, food, or alcohol with 5-HTP? Do MAO inhibitors stay in the body for a long time? How about St. John's wort? I experience a flushing sensation when taking a choline plus a vitamin B_5 product. Why? Do I have an excess of acetylcholine over serotonin? Do you think I might fare better using a 5-HTP plus St. John's wort plus a vitamin B_5 product?

DW

A: There is no problem with using an MAO inhibitor with alcohol, pain killers, or food as long as you do not have any reaction to it. I assume that you are referring to casual drinking and occasional pain killers. We cannot recommend such a 5-HTP formulation for people who abuse these substances.

Remember that everybody is biochemically different, so there is no one right answer. Generally, the half-life of an MAO inhibitor can vary from several days to several weeks. Some of the more powerful antidepressants will stay in the body longer. St. John's wort is a very mild MAO inhibitor and, therefore, I would guess that its half-life is not very long, perhaps a day or two. I couldn't find any specific data on the half-life of St. John's wort.

Choline itself can occasionally result in a mild headache, but the flush is probably from niacin. Whether you have too much acetylcholine and not enough serotonin is something that I cannot answer. You might want to experiment with the formulation that you describe and see how it makes you feel. Interestingly, all of these nutrients formulations serve to operate as boosters of your stimulus barrier. Either, or both in concert, should help you to stay asleep, and also to help you during your waking hours to move more easily between one task and another, or two tasks at the same time. Thus, they should enhance what is know "parallel processing".

WB

Serotonin Syndrome

Q: In your "Misinformation v Facts" you do not mention the sometimes fatal condition known to physicians as "serotonin syndrome" (SS) which is very similar to malignant neuroleptic syndrome.

TB

A: Serotonin syndrome is almost always the result of excessive use of either tricyclic antidepressants or SSRIs or MAO inhibitors. While Martin[1] refers to the main pathophysiologic mechanism of SS as excessive 5-hydroxytryptophan stimulation, nowhere in his research paper or in any of the literature referenced by him is there a single case of SS caused by taking 5-HTP, either alone or in combination with another agent. Some of the other contributing causal agents are LSD, MDMA, L-Dopa, lithium, buspirone, and large amounts of tryptophan. But any of these items alone are not sufficient.

It is important to note that the serotonin receptor implicated (5-HT1a) is not affected unduly or disproportionately by serotonin itself — into which 5-HTP is efficiently converted — but only when stimulation is lopsided. This means that one or a few of the HT (serotonin) receptors are disproportionately stimulated via other contributing causal agents.

At subtherapeutic levels — or the low doses used for life-extension purposes — even deprenyl (a MAO-B inhibitor) in combination with tryptophan has not been found to cause SS. Nevertheless, in spite of a paucity of adverse effects, the American manufacturer of deprenyl has recently changed the package insert to caution that there may be problems if deprenyl is used with other drugs (especially, tricyclics or SSRIs).

WB

Reference

1. Martin TG. Serotonin syndrome. *Ann Emerg Med.* 1996;28:520-526.

Best Sleep in Years with 5-HTP

Testimonial: My first before-bedtime use of 5-HTP afforded me the best night's sleep I've had in years. However, on my *second* night combining it with melatonin made me somewhat more groggy than relaxed. One reason I missed tryptophan is that it relieved both the pain and the anxiety associated with my temporal mandibular joint syndrome (TMJ). Welcome 5-HTP! Shame on the FDA!

Despite not yet having the benefit of your advice on the matter, I'm ordering acetyl glucosamine, in hopes it may favorably impact on the joint mentioned above.

By the way, that other "joint," the one never affected by arthritic disorders, certainly responds to the combination of 5-HTP and L-Arginine. If not careful, I'll get arrested!

BA

Teeth Grinding Gone with 5-HTP

Q: My wife had been a tooth grinder now for a number of years, and it's been driving me slightly crazy. I'd like to report that 5-HTP has been a godsend because since she's been taking 5-HTP her problem has gone away. What's the explanation for this?

RR

A: Nocturnal jaw clenching and grinding (also known as bruxism) are often the result of tension, anxiety, and stress which lead to jaw pain of increasing intensity and duration. It can lead to loss of teeth. Curiously, several of the SSRI's (selective serotonin reuptake inhibitors) have been found to produce bruxism.[1,2] The mechanism of SSRI-induced bruxism is unclear. A variety of theories have been proposed, including sleep disturbance, serotonergic-mediated inhibition of dopamine, manifesting as akathisia (inability to be still or at rest), and SSRI-induced anxiety. The increasingly popular recreational drug MDMA ("Ecstasy") has been found to produce bruxism in some instances possibly owing to its reported ability to damage serotonin neurons (animal studies only).[3] Tryptophan has been looked at, in at least one investigation, as a bruxism treatment, but with out beneficial results.[4] The hypothesis put forward is that there needs to be a better balance in serotonin receptor activity. While nothing has appeared in the scientific literature on 5-HTP and bruxism, we have received other reports confirming this benefit.

WB

References
1. Por CP, Watson L, Doucette D, Dolovich L. Setriline-associated bruxism. *Can J Clin Pharm*. 1996;3:123-125.
2. Romanelli F, Adler DA, Bungay KM. Possible paroxetine-induced bruxism. *Ann Pharm*. 1996;30:1246-1248.
3. McCann UD, Slate SO, Ricarte GA. Adverse reactions with 3,4-metylenedioxymethphetamine (MDMA 'ecstasy'). *Drug safety*. 1996;15:107-115.
4. Etzel KR, Stockstill JW, RUgh JD, Fisher JG. Tryptophan supplementation for nocturnal bruxism: report of negative results. *J Craniomandib Disord*. 1991;5:115-120.

How You Can Get More information

Q: Are there any research papers on 5-HTP available to the public?

EE

A: Yes. This book lists scientific references at the end of each article and these articles are not only about 5-HTP but also about other related subjects. Hard copies of these articles can be obtained through the medical library closest to your area. Most medical schools or hospitals with residency training programs have medical libraries. These references may also be obtained via Infotrieve: call 1-800-422-4633. The average paper, plus postage plus royalty, is about $15.

Other sources for finding the scientific literature on 5-HTP, as well as the multiple other subjects that *Life Enhancement* writes about, include PubMed on the web: www4.ncbi.nlm.nih.gov. /pubmed/, or the Knowledge Index from CompuServe.

Dr GV

Index

cholinergic 35
cholinergic modulation 36
chromium aspartate 119
Chronic alcohol use 95
Chronic stress 89
clinical depression 25
coagulate 25
coagulation 51, 54
cognition 37
Cognitive functions 35
cognitive impairment 37
consciousness 11
consciousness revolution 8
coronary angiography 24, 50
coronary artery bypass surgery 24, 50
coronary artery disease 24
corticotropin releasing hormone 114
cortisol 62, 89
craving 95
CRH 114
Cross-Species Aggression Control 90
CSF 91, 94
CSF 5-HIAA 94
D-fenfluramine 115
dangerous combination 95
decreased libido 112
depressed memory 37
depression 7, 15, 17, 19, 21, 23, 24, 25, 29, 31, 49, 59, 62, 65, 87, 88, 89, 94, 98
depressive disorders 17
dexamethasone 62
dexfenfluramine 83, 88, 93, 106
DHEA 105
diabetes mellitus 101
diagnostic cardiac catheterization 50
dihydroergotamine 22
Vladimir Dilman, MD, PhD, 104

get a *free* SIX-MONTH *SUBSCRIPTION*

to LIFE
enhancement

*T*his monthly newsmagazine has been hailed as the most ground-breaking in the alternative health field. It offers you the highest quality health information available anywhere at any cost. A 6-month subscription is regularly valued at $23.70 and you can get it now for *FREE!*

✔ YES, I want it!
1-800-543-3873

Simply call toll-free or send this card to get your free 6-month subscription

M ☐ F ☐

NAME   SEX

COMPANY

ADDRESS

CITY   STATE   ZIP

PHONE

Do you currently use dietary supplements?   Yes ☐ No ☐

Have you ever purchased anything by mail order?   Yes ☐ No ☐

AGE   PROFESSION

BUSINESS REPLY MAIL
FIRST CLASS MAIL PERMIT NO. 611 PETALUMA, CA

POSTAGE WILL BE PAID BY ADDRESSEE

LIVELONG PUBLISHING, INC.

POST OFFICE BOX 751390

PETALUMA, CA 94975-1390

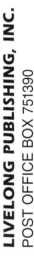